Secrets to Home Foot Care

A Practical Guide to Curing, Relieving and Preventing Foot Problems

by

Joseph W. Schneider

Character Illustrations by Lorne Silver
Diagrams by Dean Hartshorn

This book is designed to assist in dealing with common problems with the feet. The author and publisher disclaim responsibility for any adverse effects resulting from the information, programs, and management suggestions presented in this book and urge you to consult your personal physician if you have any doubts whether the treatment plan is suitable for you.

ISBN 0-9693470-0-6

Published by:
Footsaver Publishing
908 Niagara Falls Blvd.
N. Tonawanda, NY 14120-2060

DEDICATION

To my precious Amanda. At this time in your life you may only be able to eat sleep cry and soil your diapers, but you have inspired me to reach for goals I never thought attainable.

To my loving wife Sylvia. Without your everlasting strength support and guidance, I would probably be delivering pizza for a living.

ACKNOWLEDGMENTS

One man's knowledge and work rarely suffices. Projects can always be improved with the help and support of those around us.

My thanks and appreciation is extented to the following special persons whose help and contributions were included in the writing of "SECRETS TO HOME FOOT CARE".

Sylvia Schneider
Dan Haber
Vicky Wylson
Doctor Jeff Sher
Andrew Springer
Lisa Sefton
Eileen Corbet
Valmed Health Services
Esthetic & Beauty Supply
The Orthotic Group

FOREWORD

As a former professional educator in the field of disorders and treatment of the human foot, and now as a practicing foot specialist, I was pleased indeed to be asked to review this useful text. "SECRETS TO HOME FOOT CARE" gives an everyday approach and easy-to-follow insight into the cause, prevention and treatment - both self-help and professional of many common foot problems.

Much of the book's content is based upon opinions held, and methods practiced by foot health specialists throughout the world. I am hopeful that Joseph Schneider's book will reach a wide public, thereby improving the foot health of all our communities.

Roger Newell S.R.Ch.

INTRODUCTION

Dear Friend,

Feet are not glamorous or exciting. About the only time 'feet' are given any thought or consideration is after they are damaged or start hurting. Then this downtrodden, neglected part of your body screams for attention!! "SECRETS TO HOME FOOT CARE", informs you how to give your feet the care they desire. After all, who hasn't heard the old saying, "when your feet hurt, you hurt all over".

To prevent boredom, (because as I said earlier feet are not too exciting), "SECRETS TO HOME FOOT CARE", is a story about a family called "the BUNYANS". Although the names of this extended family are fictitious, they are all based on patients I have personally treated.

Together we will relive my encounters with the various Bunyans. I will tell you what treatments were administered in my office, and in a series of short, easy-to-follow instructions, how you can prevent and cure foot ailments in the comfort of your own home, without expensive doctor bills.

"SECRETS TO HOME FOOT CARE" is divided into four parts. The first part, through my interactions with the Bunyan family, discusses common foot problems, and how to cure and prevent them, in the comfort of your own home.

Part two examines diseases such as diabetes, arthritis, and gout. You will learn how they can affect the feet, and steps you can administer to control the problem.

The third part contains home exercises for the feet, that take only minutes per day. As well, there is as a very special chapter on "orthotics". Orthotics are custom made supports that fit in your shoes, which can very often cure many foot ailments.

Lastly, there is a unique chapter on "How To Constuct Foot Pads". Step-by-step instructions with accompanying diagrams, illustrate how easy it is to make foot pads to relieve painful corns, calluses, and spurs located on different areas of the feet.

You will find the answers to most of your foot problems in this book, but if there is a question you would like to ask, a form with my address is located at the back of the book. This form has space for questions, comments, or inquiries on different foot products mentioned throughout the text. I promise to answer all questions as soon as possible. Just think of me as your personal mail-order foot specialist.

Sincerely yours,

Joseph Schneider

Joseph W. Schneider B.A.A. D.Ch.

TABLE OF CONTENTS

PART 1

CHAPTER I

CHAPTER II

CHAPTER III

CHAPTER IV

CHAPTER V

Perspiring Feet

CHAPTER VI

Warts

CHAPTER VII

PART 2

CHAPTER VIII

Common Diseases That Affect The Feet

PART 3

CHAPTER IX

Foot exercises

CHAPTER X

Orthotics

PART 4

CHAPTER XI

How To Construct Foot Pads

AFTERWORD

WILEMENA BUNYAN

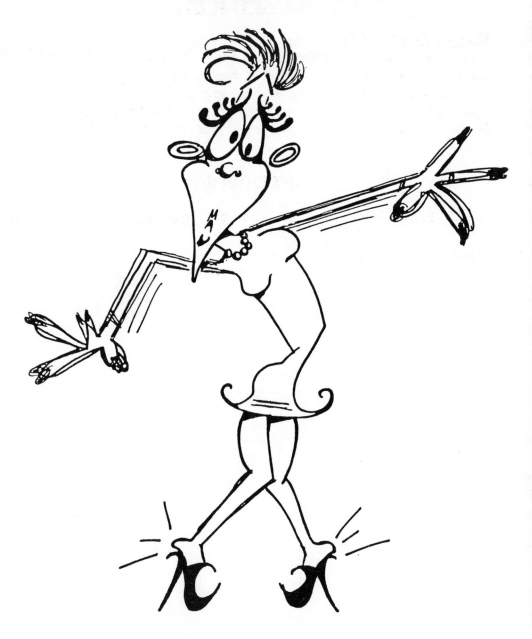

"But these are not cheap shoes, and they're so comfortable"

CHAPTER I

SHOES FOR YOU

or

"He who wears the shoes, best knows where it pinches."

It didn't seem like such a big deal at the time. It was a cold, blustery fall afternoon when Mrs. Wilemena Bunyan first limped into my office. She was attractive, about 40 years old, 5 foot 3 inches tall, with short brown hair. She was wearing pointy toe, two inch high stilleto heels. No wonder she was limping!

My secretary directed Mrs. Bunyan into my office, and I instructed her to remove her panty hose and shoes. Her feet were red and slightly swollen, with bumps on the top of her toes, corns on the side of her baby toes, and thick calluses on the soles of her feet. Not a pretty sight! I composed myself, recorded a medical history, as I do for all new patients, and casually asked her, "What is the problem with your feet?"

"My feet hurt all the time," she answered. "I've tried everything and I can't seem to get any relief."

I must tell you, I've heard that line before from many, many patients and despite what you may think, relief is possible.

The first thing I told her was that her shoes were the biggest cause of all her foot problems.

"But, these are not cheap shoes and they're so comfortable," she replied.

I've also heard that before, so it was time to give Mrs. Bunyan a brief course on the anatomy of the foot.

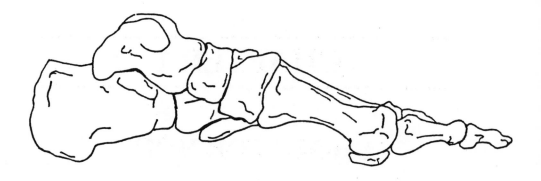

Figure 1: The AMAZING "bare to the bones" foot

The foot is one of the most complicated structures known to man. It has twenty-six small bones, fifty-six ligaments, and thirty-eight muscles. During an average lifetime a person will walk three times around the world or approximately 70,000 miles. That is a lot of walking, and with each step your foot absorbs shock, adjusts to the contours of the ground, and propels you forward, backward, upwards, downwards or sideways.

Originally, man was supposed to get help from his hands while walking, but we had to stand up. To complicate things further, man invented shoes and wore them. Too late to change that now, and besides, I don't think our knuckles could stand the scraping against the pavement.

Wilemena Bunyan was amazed at all this new information. Next I had her place her foot over the top of her high heeled, pointed toe shoes. Her foot covered the entire shoe. "You see Mrs. Bunyan," I explained, "your foot is crammed into those shoes. Without adequate room in the shoe, a great deal of chafing and pressure is caused, and that is why you get the bumps on the tops of your toes, and the corns on your baby toes. Also when you raise your heel off the ground, most of your body weight is transferred directly onto the balls of your feet, and that is why such thick calluses build up across them."

I think she understood the points I was making and asked me what could be done for her.

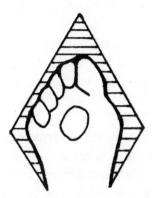

Figure 2: Crowding the toes into pointed toe shoes can lead to calluses, corns and bunions.

I gave her specific instructions on "HOW TO CHOOSE SHOES". It was perfect for her and I hope it will be useful for you too.

HOW TO CHOOSE SHOES

1) <u>Ask yourself 'for which type of activity will I wear the shoes?'</u>

Will it be for work, trips, nights on the town, shopping, special occasions or sports? For shopping or travelling the shoe should be roomy, with a firm counter and a cushioned sole. (This is especially true when going shopping for shoes.)

For sports, choose an athletic shoe that fits comfortably immediately - while you are still in the store. Most "name brands" are good but try on several different pairs before choosing. A good athletic shoe is my recommendation for all activities except maybe swimming and weddings.

Nights out or special occasion shoes are truly the scourge of mankind, especially a lady's high fashion shoe. If you must wear a fancy shoe, do so for just a few hours at a time. If possible slip them off under the table to give your feet a rest. Remember, your feet aren't pointed, so your shoes shouldn't be pointed either.

In general, you should compromise; a little less fashion for a little more comfort.

2) <u>Buy shoes late in the day.</u>

As the day wears on, feet tend to swell. To prevent the problem of shoes fitting well in the morning, but too tight at night, make your shoe purchases late in the day.

3) <u>Don't tell the salesman your shoe size.</u>

Let the salesman measure your feet in length and width while you are standing. Your foot size may change as you get older, so the size "8" that fit you at age 30 may not fit you at age 40 or 60. Also, just because your foot is measured at size "7" does not automatically mean a size "7" will fit properly. Manufacturers' sizes vary from one to the other. A size "7" of one brand may be the same as a "7 1/2" of another brand, so don't choose according to size, but according to fit.

The reason the salesman's measurement should be done while you are standing is because the foot expands while bearing weight. In other words, an active weightbearing foot is larger than a resting non-weightbearing foot. Generally the older you are, the more your foot will enlarge while standing.

Lastly, don't let a salesman put a filler in your shoe to make it fit better. Foot doctors study for years and know when your feet need extra padding; a salesperson doesn't. The shoe should fit properly on its own. A filler should only be used if there is a major size difference between your feet.

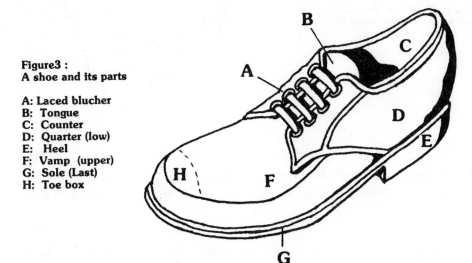

Figure3 :
A shoe and its parts

A: Laced blucher
B: Tongue
C: Counter
D: Quarter (low)
E: Heel
F: Vamp (upper)
G: Sole (Last)
H: Toe box

4) <u>What to look for in a shoe:</u>

a) Shoes should be 1/2 inch longer than your feet. While standing, press the end of your shoe to discover the position of your longest toe. Remember, the big toe is not always the longest. There should be about one finger width space between your longest toe and the end of the shoe.

b) The heel should fit snugly. If you walk around and your heel lifts out of the shoe, then the shoe is too loose.

c) Choose a shoe that is roomy in the toe area. Ideally, there should be enough room to freely wiggle your toes. Shoes that are tight in the toe area exert pressure which will cause corns, calluses, infections and nail problems, as well as dermatitis, athlete's foot and foot odor.

d) Avoid pointy-toed shoes. Your foot isn't pointed so it is only common sense to choose shoes that aren't pointed.

e) The widest part of the shoe should fit the widest part of your foot. That's the area from the big toe joint to the little toe joint.

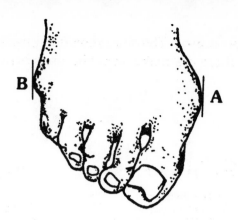

Figure 4: The widest part of your foot is from point 'A' to point 'B'. This is especially relevant if your toes are deformed or twisted towards the centre of your foot.

f) The material of the upper part of the shoe should be soft. If the material is too hard or stiff it will chafe the toes causing corns, and other toe problems. You should be able to ripple the material slightly as your finger is rolled over it from side to side.

g) Choose a shoe with a broad low heel. This kind of heel distributes your body weight properly. The higher and thinner the heel, the worse your weight is distributed, and body balance is diminished.

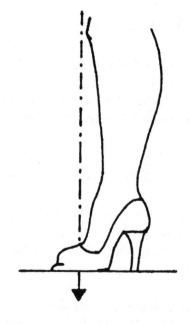

Figure 5: A thin narrow heel will cause wobbly ankles and poor balance. A high heel will shift your body weight forward onto parts of the foot not designed for carrying too much weight.

h) The shoe should bend at the sole and not the shank. A shoe that flexes at the wrong place is a sign of the upper being too stiff.

i) Check the inside of the shoe with your hand. Make sure there aren't any wrinkles, loose linings, ridges or other irregularities which could rub against the foot causing corns or blisters.

SECRETS TO HOME FOOT CARE

j) Special considerations when choosing shoes:

i) When buying sandals make sure the straps don't rub against your baby toe or the joint of the big toe. Often painful blisters occur if the straps don't suit your foot.

ii) If you regularly wear high heeled shoes, buy shoes with heels of three different heights. If you always wear heels of the same height, your calf muscles and achilles tendon will shorten. As soon as you try to wear flats, the back of your legs will hurt a great deal. If you buy shoes with flat, medium and high heels, and rotate wearing these shoes regularly, your calf muscles will remain limber and you will be comfortable in heels of all heights.

iii) If you have foot supports, take them along when shoe shopping, to make sure there is enough room for your foot and the support.

iv) If you are uncertain whether the shoe feels right, make sure it can be returned. When you get home wear them around the house for a couple of hours , or use a runway model trick. Tape the bottom of the shoes with masking tape, to prevent any visible wear. This way you can be sure that the shoes fit well.

v) Finally remember, "shoes should not be "BROKEN IN"; they are inanimate objects that will "BREAKDOWN" your feet. They may be stiff but never painful.

BERTHA BUNYAN

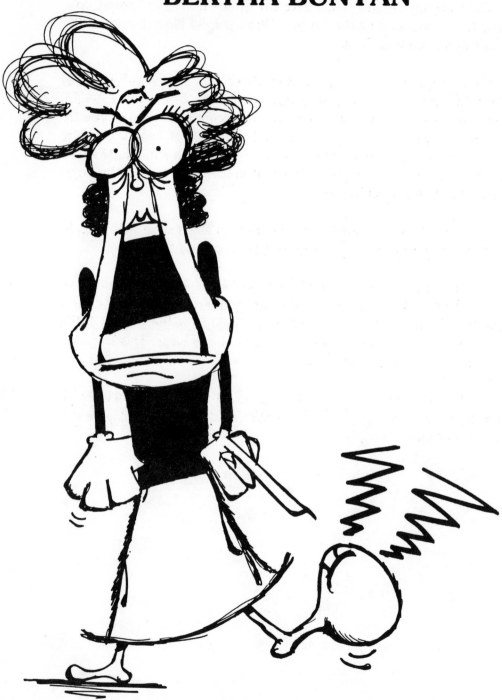

"Do Anything, Just Stop the Pain!"

SECRETS TO HOME FOOT CARE

CHAPTER II

TOENAILS

or

Special Information From My "Clipping" File

I must have made a good impression on Mrs. Bunyan because two hours after Wilemena left my office I received a call from her aunt Bertha, requesting an appointment.

Bertha Bunyan arrived four days later. She said she had ingrown toenails. This can be a very painful condition and tends to get worse if left unattended. There are different treatments for this, depending on the severity of the problem. Bertha wanted me to remove the entire nail.

"Do anything," she pleaded, "just stop the pain!"

In some cases removing the nail or just the side of the nail is the correct treatment, and this should be done only by foot doctors. A local anesthetic is injected into the toe to prevent any pain, and the doctor will remove the nail or part of the nail using special instruments. The matrix, the area from where the nail grows, can be destroyed so the nail will not grow back, or left alone depending on the doctor's judgement. Afterwards, an antiseptic cream is applied, and the toe is covered with sterile gauze, and bandaged. The patient walks away from the procedure feeling just a little discomfort or some throbbing after the anesthetic wears off. Usually, after one week the doctor will check the toe to ensure everything is OK, and send you on your way. If the matrix is not destroyed the nail will grow back. Sometimes the original problem will return, but usually there is improvement.

It might sound like the quick way to relief is to have a painful toenail removed, but the toenails and fingernails are there for a reason and should not be easily disregarded. A nail is a shield that protects the tender skin and nerve endings at the tips of the hands and feet. Your nails grow most rapidly in early childhood and, like everything else, the growth rate slows with age. The health of the nail depends on the nail bed having an adequate blood and nerve supply. When something interferes with the blood and nerve supply, toenail problems occur. Remember, if the nail is removed, you no longer have Mother Nature's shield!

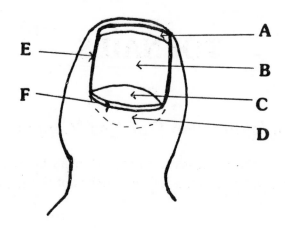

Figure 6:
A Healthy Nail and its Parts

A: The free edge (the white part of the nail)
B: The nail plate
C: The lunula (opaque 1/2 moon at the back of the nail)
D: The matrix (the area directly behind the lunula from where the nail grows)
E: The sulci (the sides where the skin and the edge of the nail meet)
F: The eponychium (cuticle)

Despite Bertha's request I was not going to remove her nails. For years she cut her toenails much too short, and as a result they had become ingrown. The big toes on both her feet were the problem areas, but any nail may be affected. This is only one of the many causes of an ingrowing nail. A complete list of the causes is found on page 12.

For Bertha Bunyan, the treatment was a lot simpler than removing her nail.

With a special nail drill, one side of her nail was trimmed to reduce the pressure. Then the sides of the nails were filed to produce a space between the edges of the nail and skin. Cotton wool was packed in the nail groove to create a protective barrier, and finally a few drops of an antiseptic called Friar's Balsam was dabbed onto the cotton wool to keep the nail groove clean and dry.

This treatment relieved Bertha Bunyan's problem, but only temporarily. To ensure that the nails didn't start hurting again, I gave her instructions to follow at home. These same instructions will help you relieve and prevent ingrown nails.

COMMON CAUSES OF INGROWING NAILS

1. Incorrect cutting of toenails: Cutting down the sides of the toenails will usually relieve a painful toe, but as the nail grows out, the problem will be worse than before. Also, a nail that is cut too short tends to curve downward and as it grows out it will push into the flesh before it reaches the edge of the toe.

2. Dropping objects on the toes: Nobody drops a frozen turkey on their toe on purpose, but when this happens, it can damage the nail causing the nail to grow incorrectly. (It also doesn't do much for the turkey.)

3. Stubbing the toes: Same as #2.

4. Improper shoes: Shoes that are too short in length, have pointy toes, or don't leave enough room in the toe box (the front part of the shoe), cause a great deal of pressure to be exerted onto the sides of the nail. This pressure will eventually cause the nail to push into the tissue surrounding the nail causing pain and tenderness.

5. Tight hosiery: Same as #4.

6. Excessive perspiration: When your feet sweat a lot, the skin around the nail becomes very soft making it easy for the nail to dig in. See chapter V on how to cure this problem.

7. Fungus infections: This is discussed further on page 23 .

8. Nutritional deficiencies: There are certain diseases such as diabetes, arthritis, obesity and others that can cause nail problems.

9. Inherited disease: This is rare and if you had an inherited nail disease you would already know about it.

PROPER NAIL CUTTING

or

"Not A Snap But Definitely A Snip"

Let the nails grow past the tip of the toe. When they get long, always cut them straight across using good nail clippers. If you have difficulty finding nail clippers, write to me and I will send you information on where you can obtain them. The proper length of the toenail, as seen in figure 7, reduces the possibility of the nail ingrowing. If you find this length too long because your nail grows too quickly, then use a file to reduce and control the length of your nail. Nail polish can beautify and hide a free edge (the white part of the end of the toenail) so that the nail will not appear too long.

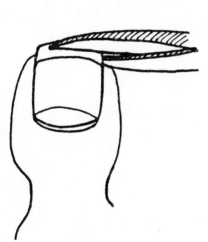

Figure 7a

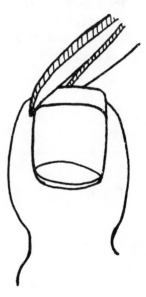

Figure 7b

Figure 7a: Correct nail cutting
Figure 7b: Incorrect nail cutting

TREATMENT FOR INGROWN NAILS

1. Soak your feet in warm soapy water for 10 minutes to soften the nails.

2. Dry thoroughly.

3. Remove the dead skin and debris in the nail groove using an orange stick.

4. Insert a wisp of sterile cotton wool using your finger or an orange stick. Do not use any sharp object to prevent cutting or marking the tender tissue.

5. Apply a drop of an antiseptic such as Betadine solution™ or Friar's Balsam™, (Tincture of Benzoine Compound). Friar's Balsam not only is a good antiseptic, but it also dries and hardens the nail groove to prevent nail penetration. This is especially good if you have perspiring feet.

6. Allow the nail to grow past the tip of the toe and replace the cotton wool as often as necessary.

BENNY BUNYAN

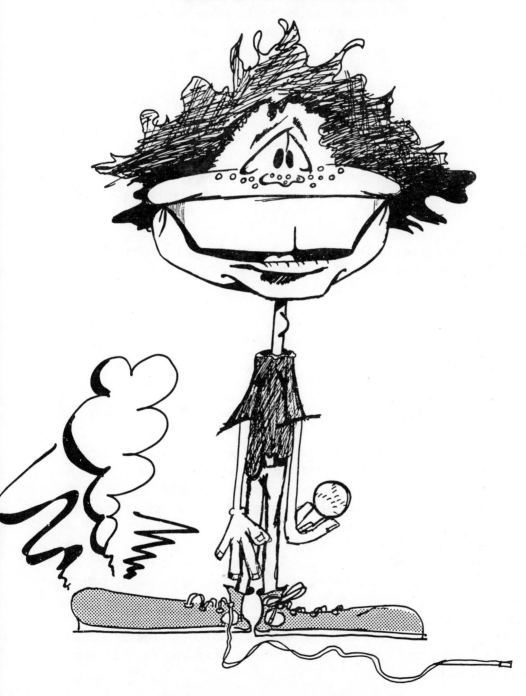

"My big toe is sort of hurting"

INFECTED TOE NAILS

I escorted Bertha Bunyan out to the reception area, and who do you think was out there waiting for her? Benny Bunyan, her 16-year-old nephew, Wilemena's son. He came to my office to give his aunt Bertha a ride home. Nice boy. As they were about to leave I told Benny to tie up the laces on his sneakers or he might trip and fall. "I can't," he answered, "my big toe is sort of hurting."
"Why don't you let me have a look at it?" I offered.
"No, it will be fine, I'm OK sir, thanks anyway."
"Benny", interjected aunt Bertha, "let the nice man look at your toe."
"No auntie, it doesn't hurt," exclaimed Benny.
"Benny!" replied aunt Bertha in a tone that was not to be denied.

Obediently, Benny Bunyan marched into my office and removed his shoes. Poor kid, I thought when I looked at his right big toe, he must be in excruciating pain.

Unlike his aunt, a sharp spike of nail from Benny's toe had penetrated the flesh. This caused a red, extremely swollen, very painful infected toe, with pus oozing out.

Teenagers going through hormonal changes in their bodies are very susceptible to ingrown toenails. However, if a person doesn't cut their nails properly, they can occur at any age.

"What have you been doing for this?" I asked Benny.
"N-nothing," he stammered.

That's not too unusual. He was just hoping the problem would go away on its own, but unless the nail penetrating the skin is removed, the toe won't heal. Also, if the toe is left untreated for a long period of time, the infection can enter the bloodstream and, in extreme cases, cause gangrene. So don't ignore an infection.

At this stage I wasn't going to do much for Benny. The toe was just too painful to touch, and until the inflammation subsided there wasn't much I could do. Some doctors would prescribe oral antibiotic pills before sending the patient home, but Benny was a healthy teenager and the instructions I gave him were good enough to reduce the infection without prescription medication. I cleaned the area with 3% hydrogen peroxide, applied a topical antibiotic and covered the toe with sterile gauze. The instructions I gave him are what you should do if you have an inflamed infected toe.

But one final word. This is not a cure for an ingrown toenail. Once the infection is reduced, let your foot specialist remove the spike of nail, don't perform minor surgery on yourself.

TREATMENT FOR AN INGROWN NAIL OR TOE INFECTION

1. Soak your foot in warm salt water. Put in enough salt so that it begins to settle on the bottom of the bowl. Soak your foot 4 times a day for no longer than 10 minutes at a time. This will drain the pus, reduce the swelling and help relieve the pain.

A few drops of 3% hydrogen peroxide will also help irrigate and cleanse the toe.

2. Carefully dry the area and apply a sterile gauze pad over the toe.

3. When the swelling has subsided, visit your foot specialist to remove the offending spike of nail.

Note: If somehow you remove the spike of nail yourself, (I don't want to know how you did it), apply a topical antibiotic on the sore area. Then, cover with a sterile gauze dressing to prevent further infection.

When Benny returned a few days later, I removed the spike along with the side of the nail then applied a topical antibiotic, and bandaged the toe.

It's like having a big thorn removed, the relief is almost instantaneous. It will be tender for a short while, but the pain will soon disappear.

GRANDMA BUNYAN

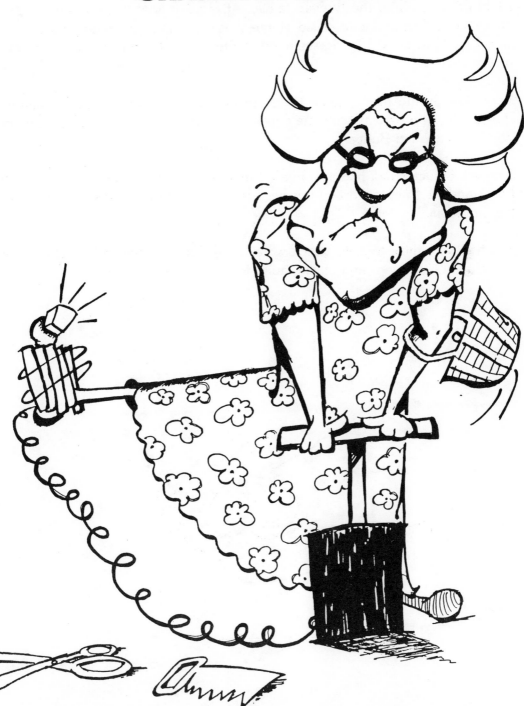

"These toenails are too thick and are difficult to cut"

THICK NAILS

I told my wife about the Bunyan family. After all, it is a little amusing having patients with foot problems called 'Bunyan'. A week and a half had gone by, but somehow I just knew I would see another Bunyan -- the family, not the growth on the foot.

Sure enough, the third patient in my office the next morning was Grandma Bunyan. My secretary just told me a new patient was coming in, she didn't mention it was another Bunyan.

She was 66 years old, had a wonderful motherly smile and told me just to call her Grandma. I never did find out her first name, because everyone just called her Grandma.

She had very thick toenails which were too difficult for her to cut. They kept snagging her stockings and poking holes in her slippers.

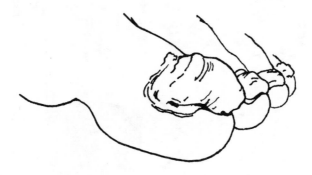

Figure 8: Thick Toenails

Thickened toenails are a problem that cannot be cured, only kept under control. I explained to Grandma Bunyan that her thick toenails were just part of the aging process. It's the same for most people. Your nails build up in layers just like skin. Every 14 days or so your top layer of skin is shed and a new layer is formed at the bottom. It's the same with nails, the top layer is shed and a new layer is formed at the nail bed. As you get older, the top layer doesn't easily shed, but the bottom layer continues to grow. As a result there is a build-up of nail, or horny skin as it is called, and as the layers accumulate the nail gets thicker and harder to cut.

I thinned the nail for Grandma Bunyan using an electric nail drill. It's completely painless and solves the problem, except that the nail will get thick again. I booked her for an appointment every two months to repeat the procedure and control the problem.

There are many other causes for thickened toenails, and if the nails are not more than 1/4" thick you can treat yourself at home.

CAUSES OF THICK NAILS

1. <u>Growing older:</u> As in Grandma Bunyan's case.

2. <u>Traumatic injury:</u> Dropping something on your toe or stubbing it may damage the matrix, the area from which the nail grows. As a result the nail will grow thick, deformed or both.

3. <u>Systemic causes:</u> If you have a problem that affects your circulation such as heart disease, a lung disorder, or peripheral vascular disease, the nails won't get proper blood nutrition and your nails will grow thick.

4. <u>Some medications</u> will cause the nails to grow thick.

5. <u>Tight shoes</u> will put pressure on the matrix which can cause thick nails.

TREATMENT FOR THICK NAILS

1. Soak your feet in warm soapy water for 10 minutes to help soften the nails.

2. Dry thoroughly.

3. Thin the nails using a good rough diamond deb file or a strong emery board. A rough diamond deb file is best.

4. If the nail is still too thick and hard, soften it further with a preparation called Whitfields ointment or a 20%-40% salicylic acid paste. Salicylic acid can burn the skin so if you have any disease such as diabetes, or peripheral vascular disease, (poor circulation), do not try this. If you do attempt this treatment, make sure the acid remains on the nail and does not touch the skin.

Even though I am telling you what you can do at home, the best treatment is to let your foot doctor thin the nail using an electric nail drill.

FUNGUS INFECTED NAILS

I think Mr. William Bunyan visited me just to meet the guy who had treated his wife, son, mother and sister. Since he was already in my office, he requested that I take a peek at his toenail which he thought had fungus on it.

He was right, he did have fungus on his toenail. He had been ignoring it because it wasn't painful or bothersome, but lately he noticed it was spreading to the adjacent toe.

"I used to play soccer for many years and often got bopped on the toe ya know. Do you think that's what caused it?"

"Could be," I answered. "Sometimes when you damage the nail, fungus will start to grow, but no one has been able to determine an exact cause for "onchomycosis", which is nail fungus. What we do know is that the nail and the nail bed provide the environment best suited for fungus. A hot, moist, dark area is home sweet home for the different parasitic fungi, yeast and molds which will grow in the nail bed."

Truthfully, I think the explanation frightened Mr. Bunyan. He just wanted me to get rid of the fungus.

For your own knowledge, I'll describe what you would see if fungus was growing on your toenails.

Fungus frequently starts growing at the front of the toenail causing the toenail to scale, then gradually becomes overgrown, pitted and blistered. Yellow streaks of powdery brittle skin and nail form, and an unpleasant odor is often present. If the nail is left unattended, it will eventually deform and the entire nail will be permanently destroyed. In severe cases, it can spread to other toes and finally, all the nails may be affected.

I'll tell you what I did for Mr. William ("just call me Bill") Bunyan in my office, and then what you can do at home.

Using an electric nail drill the nails were thinned as much as possible. With a nail probe, most of the fungus was removed. Then an anti-fungal cream to prevent new fungus from forming was applied, and the toe was covered with sterile gauze. Bill was given a prescription for an anti-fungal cream to be applied twice a day until all the fungus had disappeared. Finally, I presented him with "my home treatment for eliminating nail fungus".

MY HOME TREATMENT FOR
ELIMINATING NAIL FUNGUS

1. Soak your foot in warm soapy water for 10 minutes to soften the nails.

2. Dry thoroughly.

3. Thin the nail as much as possible using a rough diamond deb file or a strong emery board.

4. With an orange stick, remove as much of the loose powdery debris as possible.

5. Next apply an anti-fungal cream, or an anti-fungal paint.

Be patient, these treatments are effective but take several months of consistent use before the fungus is completely eliminated, depending on how badly the nails are infected. I repeat, you must be patient and persistent.

6. Sterilize your shoes with an anti-fungal agent. Shoes provide an excellent environment for fungal growth, and are never thoroughly cleaned inside. Fungal spores can live in the shoes and continually infect and re-infect your feet, so it is important to get tough with these organisms that hide in your shoes.

To sterilize the shoes, place them in a plastic bag or sealed box along with some sponges soaked in formaldehyde. The formaldehyde which is trapped in the sealed container will destroy the fungus, or bacteria, and their spores without harming the shoes.

There is also a prescription oral medication against nail fungus which is taken daily. It is called "Griseofulvin" and is usually taken for 10 months to a year before results appear, but it's not always successful. This is usually prescribed for someone who has fungus infections in all of their nails. Your foot specialist or family doctor is the best person to ask if this treatment would be suitable for you.

There are over 90 different toenail diseases. I've just mentioned the most common ones. If you have a nail problem that I have not mentioned, and wish to know what you can do for your specific problem, complete and send me the form at the back of the book.

WINNIFRED CRATCHET

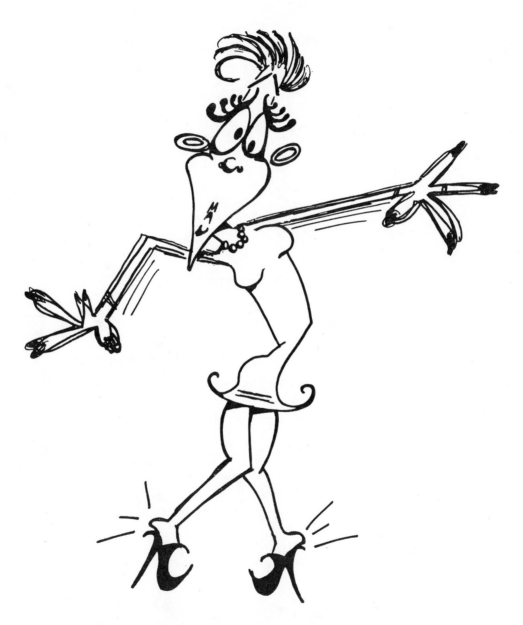

"Sometimes I feel as if my feet are on fire"

SECRETS TO HOME FOOT CARE

CHAPTER III

CALLUSES

or

Great "Balls" Of Fire

The next morning when I arrived at my office, Wilemena Bunyan was waiting for me. At least, at first glance, I thought it was Wilemena, but I was wrong. Of course this wasn't the first time I've been wrong about something, and certainly not the last time either. It was Wilemena's unmarried twin sister Winnifred Cratchet.

"I hope you don't mind my dropping by without an appointment, but I've been most anxious to see you," she exclaimed.

"No I don't mind at all Miss Cratchet," replied, "please come right in."

After all, by this time I was almost a folk hero to the Bunyans, how could I possibly refuse.

Winnifred's feet, like the rest of her, were identical to her sister. Her major complaint were the thick "burning" calluses across the balls of her feet.

"Sometimes I feel as if my feet are on fire," she uttered, as a pained look crossed her face.

"Burning feet, as you call it, can be a result of a few things. If the blood circulation to your feet is poor, then you may get the burning sensation. Or thick callus on the balls of your feet may cause them to burn."

There are a few things which I'll list later that can be done to help relieve the burning.

Winnifred's calluses were due to poor footwear.

As I explained to Winnie Cratchet, "callus is dry, hard, yellowish skin that usually appears across the ball of the foot or around the heels. When there is excess pressure or friction on the skin, the body will defend itself by laying down extra layers of skin to protect the bones and soft tissue underneath. As long as the pressure continues, more and more layers of hard skin is formed. If the pressure is removed, or redistributed, the callus will diminish or disappear."

Miss Cratchet liked to wear high heels. A normal, dainty, little foot placed in a high heeled shoe is thrust forward in the shoe. An abnormal amount of weight is transferred onto the balls of the feet, causing calluses to develop. Buying proper shoes was the best long term advice I could give Winnie.

The reason her feet were burning was directly due to the calluses. They were so thick and hard across the ball of her foot that the skin lost its elasticity. That means that the skin was totally inflexible and unable to stretch normally while she was walking, causing hot burning feet.

I had Winnie soak her feet in warm water for about 10 minutes to soften the skin and stimulate the circulation. Then I pared down the thick inflexible callus with a sharp scalpel (knife). Removing the callus returned flexibility to the skin relieving the problem. Lastly, I applied a 1/4" cushioned pad to protect the area and to prevent any soreness when she walked out of my office. Cushioned and felt pads are a very important part of your home care plan. See chapter XI for full details on how to construct your own foot pads.

Another method of redistributing the weight on your feet properly to prevent calluses are with foot orthotics. These are customized foot supports which fit in your shoes to rebalance your feet. Orthotics are a very important part of overall foot care and I will discuss them in more detail in chapter X.

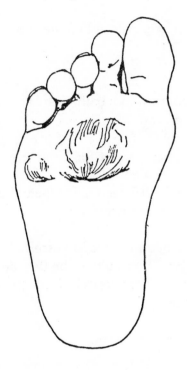

Figure 9: Callus Buildup across the Ball of the Foot

After I finished Winnifred Cratchet's treatment, she literally started dancing in my office.

"Oh Joseph, how can I ever repay you, I feel like a new woman."

"This is only the start," I explained to her, there are things you can do at home to help with the burning sensation, and to reduce the chance of reforming callus. I re-emphasized that if she continued wearing the same shoes the thick calluses and burning would surely return. She assured me that she would follow all my instructions to the letter!!

I gave her two separate fact sheets. The first was "How to relieve burning feet", and the second was "How to reduce calluses".

HOW TO RELIEVE BURNING FEET

or

"Cooling those Great Balls of Fire"

There are two methods which help relieve burning feet:

1. Contrast Footbaths

Two bowls are needed for a contrast foot bath. One filled with warm to hot water, the other filled with cold water from the tap.

    i) Place your feet in the warm water for 1 minute.

    ii) Then in the cold water for 15 seconds. Repeat the process 4 times, finishing with your feet in the warm water.

The warm water will dilate or open the blood vessels. The cold water will constrict or close the blood vessels. The result will be the stimulation of the circulation, by opening then closing the blood vessels. Once the blood is flowing freely the burning sensation disappears.

Contrast foot baths are also very useful for:

a) Relieving foot aches and pains at the end of the day. This is especially good if you stand all day or wear constricting shoes to the office.

b) Rejuvenating tired feet. Especially good for senior citizens whose feet get tired after walking short or long distances.

c) Reducing foot strain and congestion. For people who have imbalanced walking patterns due to foot, leg or back problems.

d) Stimulating blood circulation. For people with hot, burning feet.

The other method to relieve burning feet is:

2. Apply a Cooling Lotion or Cream

A cooling lotion or cream will directly relieve burning and many of the creams have ingredients that will help stimulate blood flow.

Finally, counteracting the burning sensation will only provide you with short term relief. The best long term answer is to reduce or eliminate the callus.

REDUCING CALLUS AT HOME

1. Soak your feet in warm soapy water for 10 minutes to soften the callus. (Note: soaking for longer than 10 minutes will dry out the skin on your feet).

2. Callus can also be softened by using a 1% solution of potassium hydroxide or bicarbonate of soda, but warm soapy water is easiest.

3a. Rub at the thick hardened skin using a rough turkish towel, pumice stone or a chiropody sponge. This will quickly and safely remove layer after layer of callus restoring some of the skin's elasticity. OR

3b. Apply a sloughing lotion to the hard dry skin. The cream will penetrate the callus and by just rubbing with your hands, the callus will begin to flake away.

The best time to try to remove calluses is right after bathing. If you just do it sporadically it won't help much. It is best to make "removing calluses" part of your daily bathing routine, and you will easily be able to control the problem.

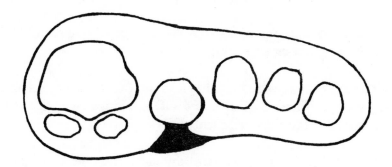

Figure 10: A Cross-section of a Dropped Metatarsal Head, with Callus Formation under the Bone

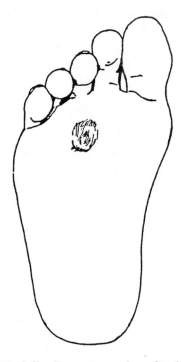

Figure 11: Callus Formation under a Single Metatarsal Head.

MORE ON CALLUSES

Another type of callus forms under one or two bones on the bottom of the feet. These bones are called metatarsals, and calluses that form under the head of the metatarsal are due to abnormal pressure or improperly balanced feet.

This was the situation with Carrie (Gram) Cratchet, Winnie and Wilemena's mother. She suffered from terrible osteo-arthritis and her 3rd metatarsal bone dropped below the level of the other metatarsals. Due to this, more weight than the bone was designed to carry was placed over that single area. The skin was bruised and irritated, with a very painful callus. Also a corn was in the middle of the callus where most of the weight was concentrated.

Treating this type of callus at home is the same as I have previously described, but to rid yourself of the problem, your body weight must be distributed over the bottom surface of your feet. Felt or cushioned padding will help you achieve this goal. See Chapter XI.

The best devices to rebalance the foot, properly distribute body weight, eliminate or reduce calluses and corns, are foot orthotics.

AND EVEN MORE ON CALLUSES

Causes of heel calluses are: sling back shoes, hard sandals, but mostly dryness. In severe cases the dryness is so bad that the skin cracks, and deep fissures develop all around the heel.

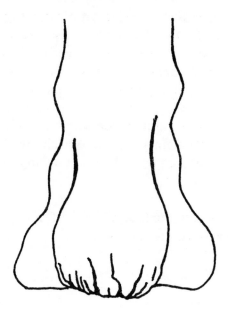

Figure 12: A Dry Cracked Fissured Heel

TREATMENT FOR DRY CALLUSED HEELS

or

Patient "Heel" Thyself

The only treatment is to reduce the callus, and restore moisture to the skin.

A) <u>Reducing callus:</u>

1. Soak your feet in warm soapy water.

2. Using a chiropody sponge, pumice stone, or rough file, rub away as much of the dry skin as possible.

3. Apply a good sloughing lotion to flake away dry callus.

4. Apply a good moisturizing cream.

B) <u>Restoring moisture to the skin:</u>

1. Before going to sleep, apply a moisturizing cream around the heels. Cover it with a plastic wrapping through the night.

2. In the morning, repeat the procedure for reducing callus.

NOTE: You will find many good moisturizing creams on the market. One that I have found to be excellent, especially for dry cracked heels, is an old remedy called "Balsam of Peru". Ask your pharmacist if he/she will prepare a jar in paste form, for you to try. (It will be much cheaper if you can find a pharmacy that already has the mixture prepared.)

GRANDPA BUNYAN

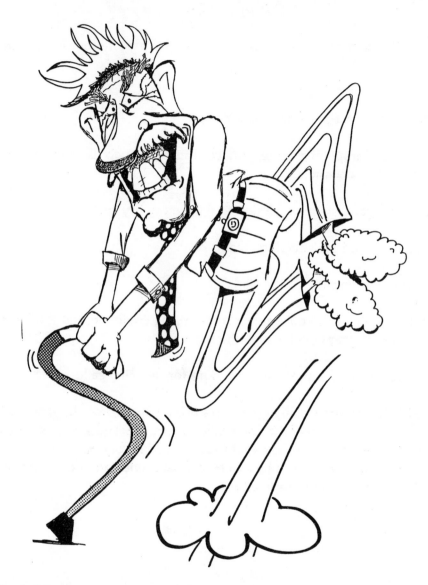

"I feel 20 years younger, that would make me only 80."

CHAPTER IV

CORNS

or

Hell hath no fury like a "woman's corn"

Grandpa Bunyan strolled into my office one afternoon. He was a tall, thin man about 68 years old with a full head of long graying hair. He leaned on his cane, looked down at me and said, "Son, what do you do with corns?"

I gazed up into his eyes and sincerely replied, "Usually I boil it in salt water for about 5 to 10 minutes, then liberally spread butter over it, add a sprinkling of salt and eat it right off the cob."

For about 10 seconds silence penetrated the office, then Grandpa Bunyan let out a bellow of laughter that shook the walls. He slapped me on the back, knocking me forward three feet and above his chuckling said, "C'mon son I want you to take a gander at my feet." That meant have a look at his feet.

His toes were bent out of shape causing him to have several really nasty corns.

"What d'ya think of them?" he said, as if he was proud of his corns, "they hurt like the dickens!".

"To tell you the truth," I answered, "if I had to choose I'd prefer the corn on the cob."

That started wave upon wave of laughter. Between you and me, it wasn't such a funny line, but I think he just enjoyed life and laughter.

This was a man I instantly liked and I wanted to do all I possibly could to help him. He had two corns on the tips of his 3rd and 4th toes on his right foot, and a corn on the top of the 2nd toe on his left foot. I explained to him that a corn was a growth of very hard cone shaped skin, caused by friction or pressure on a specific part of the foot. He then pointed to the corn on his 2nd toe and said, "would you believe son, that I kin tell ya the weather because of that little b........."

I believed him. How many times have you or a friend of yours been able to predict the weather because of a corn? Well it's true, a corn can be your own private barometer. Often corns occur over joints, and the point of the cone shaped corn can reach deep into the joint causing bursitis. A bursae is a fluid-filled sac that lubricates the joints and when a corn invades this sac, painful inflammation occurs, called bursitis. With the approach of bad weather, the outdoor atmospheric pressure drops. This causes the bursa, which is already inflamed due to the corn, to fill with even more fluid. This excess fluid stimulates and expands the tissue surrounding the joint, creating greater pressure and more pain. And that allows the accurate prediction of the onset of bad weather.

I soaked Grandpa Bunyan's feet in warm water to soften the corns and proceeded to cut off the offending corns with a scalpel. Afterward I applied special pads to protect and deflect pressure away from the sore areas.

He left my office with a wide smile on his face, winked at my secretary, and said, "I feel 20 years younger, that would make me only 80."

All the way down the hall we could hear him laughing at his own joke. What a guy!.

The type of pad I made for Grandpa Bunyan is one that you can easily construct for yourself (see chapter XI). Home treatment for corns varies, depending on where they appear on the foot. The next four sections are divided according to the area where a corn can appear on your feet.

CORNS ON THE TOPS OF THE TOES

or in your case

A cause for "corn-cern"

Corns on the tops of the toes are always a result of the shoe rubbing against the joint of the toe. Usually they are caused by poorly fitting shoes, or by malformed feet or toes.

TREATMENT

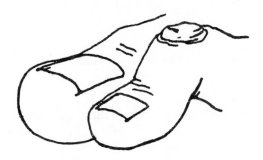

Figure 13: A Corn on the top of a Hammer Toe

1. The best solution is to purchase shoes with a large toe box so that the shoe doesn't rub on the toes.

2. An alternative to this is to stretch the shoe in the area that is rubbing, or cut away part of the shoe to relieve the pressure.

3. A felt pad in the shape of a crescent placed behind the corn will deflect the shoe pressure away from the corn and onto the pad. Detailed instructions for this pad are found on page 99. Felt or cushioned padding are the best materials for this, but if you don't have any handy, a piece of folded over gauze placed behind the corn will deflect pressure away from the sore spot.

4. The last and worst treatment for corns on the tops of the toes comes under the heading of "BATHROOM SURGERY". This is when you cut the corn off yourself. I don't recommend this because the possibility of infection when you treat yourself is very high. It is best to see a foot specialist who can remove the corn safely, but if you cut off the corn yourself, like so many people do, follow these instructions:

a) Soak your foot in warm soapy water to clean and soften the corn.

b) Dry the area thoroughly.

c) Try using a pumice stone or chiropody sponge to reduce the corn before you use a knife.

d) If this hasn't worked, sterilize the area with a 70% solution of isopropyl alcohol.

e) With a sterilized sharp knife or razor blade snip off **just the top** of the hard dead skin.

f) Next apply a topical antiseptic over the area where you cut off the corn.

g) Protect the corn with padding as described earlier, or use moleskin, a thin felt adhesive padding, or tubefoam, foam shaped like a tube which fits directly over the toe.

If you do happen to snip too much skin off and cut yourself, pack the area with sterile cotton or sterile gauze and apply pressure to stop the bleeding. Afterwards, administer a topical antibiotic cream on the area, and cover with a sterile gauze or bandage. Immediate action will help prevent infection.

One final word of warning. DO NOT USE CORN PLASTERS. Corn plasters contain acid that can burn the healthy skin as well as the dead hard tissue. Corn plasters often cause small sores or ulcers and should be avoided.

CORNS AT THE TIPS OF THE TOES

Corns at the tips of the toes are sometimes caused by wearing short shoes, but usually they are a result of deformed toes. The angle of the toe in relation to the ground causes it to take pressure with every step, and therefore a corn develops.

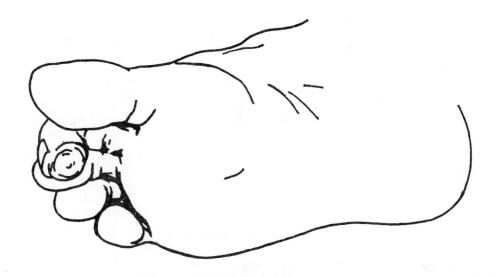

Figure 14: A Corn at the Tip or Apex of the 2nd Toe

TREATMENT

1. The best way to prevent and cure this problem is to cut a felt pad and wedge it under the offending toe or toes. Instructions for this type of pad can be found on page101. If you don't have any felt, just about any soft material wedged under the toe will do. The pad will lift the toe off the ground eliminating the pressure and the problem.

2. To cut the hard skin, follow the same instructions described in "Treatment for corns on the tops of the toes".

CORNS BETWEEN THE TOES

Corns between the toes are called soft corns because the moisture between the toes makes them soft and rubbery. Soft corns are caused by the toes rubbing against one another due to tight shoes, or malformed feet with oddly shaped toes.

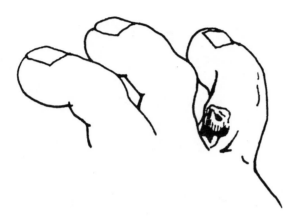

Figure 15: A Corn between the Toes

TREATMENT

To eliminate a soft corn the toes must be kept a) dry and b) separated.

1. To keep moisture out from between the toes, make sure you dry thoroughly after bathing. If that isn't enough apply a light coating of talcum powder, or isopropyl alcohol or any other suitable drying agent.

2. To prevent the friction which causes the soft corns, separate the two toes using a piece of lambs wool, moleskin, cotton wool or a small felt or cushioned pad. Instructions for this pad can be found on page 103.

CORNS ON THE SOLES OF THE FEET

Corns on the soles of the feet are caused by an imbalanced foot where one area, usually the head of a metatarsal, absorbs too much pressure resulting in corn formation. See figures 10 & 11.

TREATMENT

1. Treatment is the same as the treatment for a callus on the sole of the foot, found on page 92.

2. Relieve the pressure and distribute the weight by making a foot pad. Construction of pads are found on pages 89 through 96.

3. Orthotics. Check chapter X.

INFECTED CORNS

You should not attempt to cut an infected corn. If the corn is hot, red, swollen and pus is evident, you should just try to reduce the infection.

TREATMENT

1. Soak the foot in warm salt water. Add enough salt to the water so that it begins to accumulate on the bottom of the bowl. This will help reduce the inflammation and drain some of the pus.

2. Apply a non-prescription antibiotic ointment and cover with a sterile gauze or bandage.

3. If the inflammation doesn't subside see your foot or family doctor.

MINIMAL INCISION SURGERY

Approximately 40% of all patients who visit my office do so because of a pain-ful corn. I have related several home treatments for the different kinds of corns. If you have tried my suggestions and you're still unsuccessful at eliminating the corns, there is a quick, painless surgical technique that can help you. It is called "MINIMAL INCISION SURGERY" and is performed at your podiatrist's office or the hospital. This procedure can permanently remove corns, and when it is over you walk away from the table. Just one word of caution, it is expensive. If you're still interested, contact your podiatrist for further details.

BOBBY BUNYAN

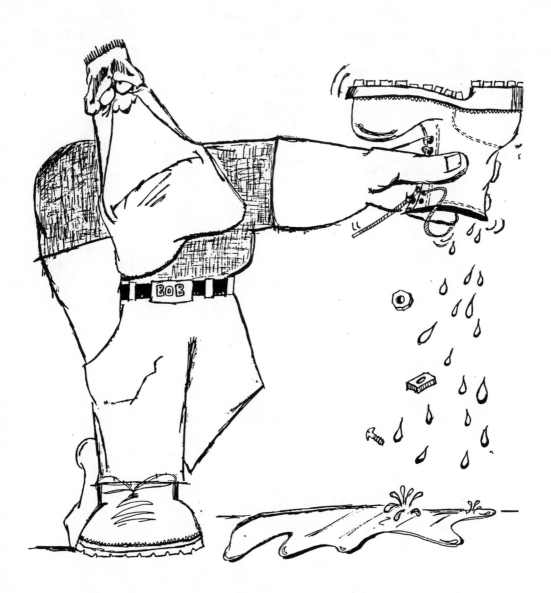

*"When Bobby took off his shoes the smell was so bad
it made my eyes water"*

SECRETS TO HOME FOOT CARE

CHAPTER V

PERSPIRING FEET

Several weeks had passed before I heard again from Wilemena Bunyan. She called during my lunch one day to frantically ask if I could help her brother-in-law.

"What's the problem?," I asked.

"It's his feet. Bobby came over for dinner last night and when he took off his shoes, the smell nearly made me faint. I was embarassed, he was humiliated and the whole evening was ruined. Is there any way to help him?"

I thought she was exaggerating and I assured her I could help her brother-in-law.

His work in construction was very seasonal and he didn't want to lose any time off work, so I told him to come in the following week at the end of his shift.

Bobby Bunyan was 38 years old, a tall stocky, very well built man. I politely asked him to remove his construction boots and socks. He sheepishly looked at me and said, "Ya sure you want me to do that? Could ya just give me some instructions like ya did for the others?"

"I will," I replied, "but let me check over your feet anyway."

There are not too many hazards in my profession, but when Bobby took off his shoes, I wanted to apply for combat pay. The smell was so bad it made my eyes water, but I couldn't let him know that I was disturbed. He was embarrassed enough already. I composed myself and immediately had him soak his feet.

The first thing I needed to do was to assure him that he did not stink. He suffered from a medical problem that was not his fault and it could be corrected.

As his feet were soaking I explained, "There are more sweat glands on the palms of your hands and the soles of your feet than any other part of your body. You seldom hear anyone complain of smelly hands, because hands are exposed to the air, and the moisture is able to evaporate. Unlike hands, feet are constricted by shoes and socks. When feet perspire, the moisture cannot easily evaporate. Sweaty feet is a condition medically known as 'HYPERHIDROSIS'. Sweaty feet alone is not why feet have an odor. When the moisture on the feet, especially between the toes, accumulates, bacteria and fungus will start to grow. Bacteria and fungus love a warm dark moist place in which to multiply, and it is the build up of bacteria and fungus on the feet that cause the foul foot odor. Medically this is called 'Bromidrosis'."

Bobby dried his feet and then, feeling a little better knowing it wasn't his fault, allowed me to check his feet. With the moisture and bacteria cleaned away his feet no longer had any odor, but he had other problems which will afflict a person whose feet perspire profusely. On the ball of his feet and his heels he had a multitude of tiny blisters, and between his toes the skin was all macerated. That means white, rubbery and flaky. I painted some 1% gentian violet between his toes to help dry out the maceration and applied a weak solution of 1% iodine to help the skin absorb the small blisters. Then I sprinkled a special powder on his feet which would help reduce the amount of sweating and slow down the growth of bacteria. That was really all I could do for him in my office.

"The rest is up to you, Bobby," I told him as I issued him an instruction sheet to follow at home. If he was going to eliminate his problem, he would have to make this part of his daily routine.

To make things a little easier for you, I will expand and divide the instructions into five parts. a) Causes, b) Treatment - 3 stages, c) Complications, d) A Special Doctor's Treatment, e) A brief summary.

CAUSES OF FOOT PERSPIRATION AND FOOT ODOR

1. <u>Hard work:</u> This is normal and healthy, but if your body and your feet sweat, a problem occurs when the moisture accumulates on your feet.

2. <u>Tired or strained feet:</u> People who stand all day, walk on hard surfaces, wear constricting boots or shoes, or have improperly balanced feet (for example deformed or flat feet) have a tendency to experience a great deal of foot perspiration.

3. <u>Mental or environmental stress:</u> When you are nervous, or worried about something, you may notice that your hands get hot and clammy. Meanwhile down at the other end of your body, the same thing is happening to your feet. Also, someone who is fretting over having bad foot odor is causing emotional stress which will only increase the problem.

4. <u>A disturbance in the nervous system or a body disorder:</u> Some diseases such as anaemia will lower your body's resistance to disease and can lead to excess sweating.

5. <u>Ingestion of certain foods:</u> Foods with powerful odors such as onions, garlic or pepper may be contributing factors to foot odor. Sometimes just altering your diet may help the problem.

TREATMENT FOR SWEATY FEET—IN THREE STAGES

1. REDUCE THE FLOW OF SWEAT SECRETED BY THE SWEAT GLANDS.

To reduce the flow of sweat, the strain and congestion of the feet must be relieved.

a) Contrast foot baths: As described on page 30.

b) Dry the feet thoroughly after bathing, preferably using a rough towel. This will dry the feet and help stimulate circulation.

c) Mechanical relief of foot strain: Imbalanced feet cause a great deal of strain on the feet, legs and back. This strain frequently causes the feet to sweat. Relief is obtained by properly aligning the feet through the use of foot orthotics. Properly balanced feet allow the feet and lower limb to function most efficiently, reducing the strain on the feet. More on orthotics can be found in chapter X.

d) Exercise: Exercise stimulates circulation and helps restore proper muscular tone. A list of foot exercises are found in chapter IX.

2. PREVENTING ACCUMULATION OF SWEAT ON THE FEET

This stage is the most important for preventing sweaty feet and foot odor.

a) Personal hygiene: Wash your feet every day, thoroughly drying between the toes using a rough towel.

b) Aeration: Aeration means allowing the sweat to evaporate. To do this there must be a flow of air around the skin.

    i) The best solution is to sit in the fresh air with your feet exposed to the air. I'm sure that this is the treatment everyone would love to do, but it is not practical during the winter, or if you work for a living.

    ii) In the summer, wear sandals without socks or stockings. With the feet exposed to the air the moisture can evaporate.

    iii) Always wear shoes constructed of porous materials such as leather. Shoes made of rubber, plastic or vinyl suffocate your feet causing them to sweat even more than usual.

iv) Alternate your footwear on a daily basis. Sweat will collect in your shoes and as described on page 24, shoes provide an excellent environment for the growth of bacteria and fungus, which are the main culprits in producing foot odor. Changing your shoes every day will not only give them a chance to dry after each wearing, but will also prolong the life and appearance of each pair of shoes.

v) Sterilize your shoes. To kill existing fungal spores and bacteria that already live in your footwear, sterilize your shoes. It is a quick and easy procedure which can be found on page 24.

vi) During the day take your shoes off whenever possible. This will give your feet a chance to breathe and flexing your foot muscles feels good. Try it, you'll like it.

c) Hosiery: Both shoes and socks absorb some of the sweat from your feet. I've already discussed shoes, so the next important item is hosiery. Socks that are capable of absorbing moisture should always be worn.

Cotton socks are the best, as well as the most comfortable. All wool socks or a wool-synthetic mixtures are also good. Nylon socks are bad and nylon stockings are the very worst. Nylon stockings for women are the biggest contributor to sweaty, smelly feet. My ears are buzzing. Women all over North America are asking, "How do you expect us to wear a dress without nylon stockings?" Unfortunately, I don't have the answer to that question, but as Sergeant Friday would say, "I'm relating the facts Ma'am, just the facts."

Finally change your socks daily, and more often if your feet perspire excessively.

3. INCREASING THE SKIN'S RESISTANCE TO SWEATING

The last stage in the treatment of sweaty feet is to apply different preparations on your feet to help reduce sweating.

Some drying agents available in your drug store are:

i) Isopropyl alcohol or surgical spirit.
ii) Calamine lotion.
iii) Hammamelis water. This is useful if your feet are inflamed.

Drying agents should be followed with the use of:

iv) Dusting powder: Dusting powders do not absorb sweat, but act as lubricants reducing the amount of friction on the feet. Many contain ingredients to help destroy fungus and bacteria. Ask your pharmacist to help you choose a dusting powder for feet. Another useful product is flat insoles that are placed inside your shoe. They have a limited life span, but do help in absorbing some moisture and foot odor.

COMPLICATIONS DUE TO SWEATY FEET

Perspiration on the feet can cause other minor problems which you can easily treat at home.

1. <u>Maceration and fissures between the toes</u>: Moisture between the toes causes the skin to turn white, and become rubbery and flaky. Often the skin will crack and bleed and an infection can set in. To prevent this, the skin between the toes must be kept dry. Applying 1% gentian violet paint, or Friars Balsam, both antiseptics, will dry and heal the area between the toes.

2. <u>Blisters and inflammation</u>. Sweat on the soles of the feet can cause many small blisters over the balls of the feet and/or the heels. Also there may be some general inflammation.

    i) For closed blisters; apply a weak iodine solution over the blisters to help absorb the fluid in the skin.

    ii) For open blisters; apply an antiseptic cream and sterile gauze.

    iii) For inflammation; soak your feet in hammamelis water (available at most drug stores) to help reduce the inflammation and soothe the feet.

SPECIAL DOCTOR'S TREATMENT
FOR SWEATY FEET

Despite all the instructions I have just given you, there are times when no amount of home care can help. Cheer up, doctors now have a special treatment, used to control excessive foot sweating called "IONTOPHORESIS".

A low frequency electric current is transmitted through a solution in which the feet are soaking. This "electric plating" of the feet, reduces the amount of foot perspiration and diminishes the chances of fungus infection. Each application can last up to six weeks at a time and is available for home care.

Also available is a special cream to fight the growth of bacteria or fungus on the feet. This cream will not stop foot sweat but will eliminate foot odor from 7-14 days after each application.

For more information on these treatments, please send the form at the back of the book.

BRIEF SUMMARY FOR TREATMENT
OF SWEATY FEET

Your daily routine should consist of:

1. Regular bathing of the feet.

2. Careful and thorough drying with a rough towel.

3. Alternating footwear each day.

4. Changing socks at least once a day after washing and drying the feet.

5. Application of a drying agent.

6. Using a dusting powder in the socks and on the feet.

Additional products that can help reduce sweat.

7. Foot orthotics to balance the feet and lower limb.

8. Inserting odor absorbing insoles in the shoes.

9. Application of Anti-Smell foot cream.

10. Use of a special appliance to reduce sweating for 6 week periods.

BONITA BUNYAN

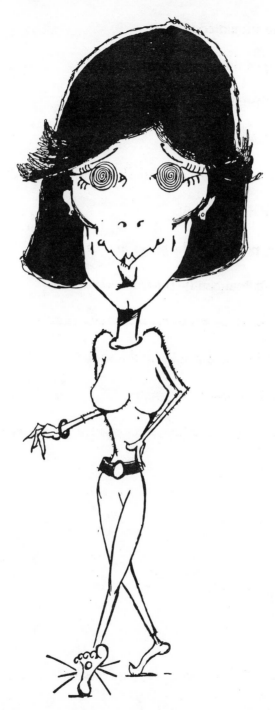

"How in the world did I get a wart?"

CHAPTER VI

WARTS

When Wilemena's daughter Bonita visited me, I just froze. Bonita Bunyan was so beautiful she literally took my breath away, but anyone can have foot problems.

Bonita complained of a corn on the sole of her foot. I took a closer look at her foot, and although it looked like there was a hard corn near her 3rd metatarsal head, I wasn't sure. With a scalpel I reduced some of the callus covering the suspected "corn". The normal striations or lines on the bottom of her foot detoured around the "corn" instead of going through it, and I presumed it wasn't a corn at all, but a plantar wart. There is one sure way of finding out. If you push on a corn it will hurt, but on a plantar wart, if you squeeze the sides of the wart it will elicit excruciating pain. I warned Bonita that I was going to squeeze the growth and it might hurt. From the scream she let out, my presumption was confirmed; it was a wart not a corn.

"How in the world did I get a wart?" she asked.

I explained to her, "Nobody really knows what causes warts, but I can tell you for sure that touching a toad with your bare hands does not cause them." She gave me a warm, captivating smile as I continued.

"A wart is a virus. Plantar warts are most often spread in places where people walk around barefoot, like swimming pools or health clubs". I asked Bonita if she belongs to a health club, and she nodded her head.

"To prevent catching another plantar wart always wear rubber sandals around public pools or in health clubs. For the time being, cover your wart with moleskin or colorless nailpolish to prevent sharing it with others, because warts can be very contagious."

"I thought warts were bumps on the skin," Bonita commented sweetly.

"On the hands or any other skin surface they are," I replied, "but a plantar wart or "verrucae" as it is medically called, is pushed down into the skin from the pressure of walking on it. It is called a plantar wart, because it is located on the plantar surface of the foot. Since it is deep under the skin it can be very difficult to get rid of it."

There are three different ways to combat plantar warts:

1. Hyfrecation: An electric wire with a specialized electric current is used to burn off the wart.

2. Chemical treatments: Application of acid directly on the wart for a period of 4 to 10 weeks, usually works very well. Many foot specialists use this method, but it means the patient must return every week for a long time before the wart disappears completely.

Chemical treatments are the best method for home care wart removal, for which I will later provide step-by-step instructions.

3. Cryotherapy: Using a special machine, the wart is destroyed by freezing its cells. This method is quickest and most effective. Often the wart is killed in one to three applications of the freezing agent. I used cryotherapy to rid Bonita Bunyan of the wart on her foot.

To eliminate the wart at home there are some things of which you must be aware. There are two different kinds of warts most often found on the foot.

A) A plantar wart which Bonita Bunyan had: This wart usually appears pearly white, soft, and may have little black specks in it. These specks are tiny blood vessels, and if you attempt to cut the wart with a knife or razor, they will bleed a great deal. Often they are mistaken for corns and can have an overlying layer of callus covering them.

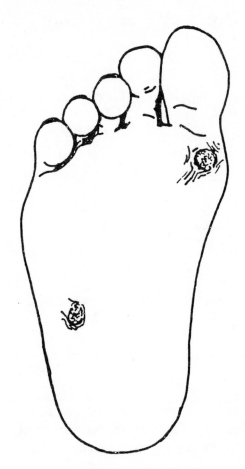

Figure 16: A Plantar Wart

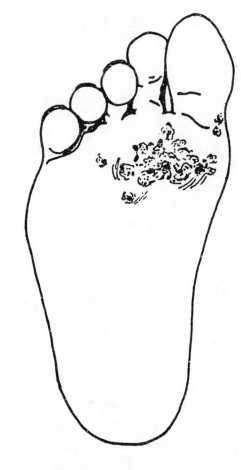

Figure 17: A Mosaic Wart

B) A mosaic wart: These warts appear as multiple flat, white circles spread over a large area. Often it will cover the entire heel, or the ball of the foot. It is rarely painful, but because it covers a large surface of the foot, it is best if your foot specialist provides treatment.

Both types of warts are contagious, so don't touch them with your hands and change your socks daily.

Sometimes, you can pass the warts from one foot to the other by switching contaminated socks. To prevent passing your wart to someone else in your family or at a public pool or club, always keep the wart covered.

TREATMENT FOR REMOVAL OF A PLANTAR WART

or

How to avoid becoming a "Worry-Wart"

Note: If you are a diabetic or have peripheral vascular disease DO NOT use acid on your feet. In other words, this treatment is not for you. If you are not sure, check with your family doctor first before using this home care treatment.

1. Soak your foot in warm soapy water for 10 minutes.

2. Dry thoroughly.

3. Use a chiropody sponge or a pumice stone to remove the callus covering the wart.

4. Cut a small oval pad 1/4" or 1/8" thick which will cover the wart, but do not stick the pad on your foot.

5. Cut a hole slightly larger than the size of the wart, and adhere the pad to the foot with the opening over the wart. This pad will transfer the body pressure away from the wart, and help push the wart towards the surface of the skin.

6. a) Cut a piece of salicylic acid plaster the exact size of the wart and apply it to the skin. This plaster is filled with 20% to 40% salicylic acid and is available in most drug stores in packages containing small sheets. Those sheets can simply be cut with scissors.

When you apply the plaster to your foot, make sure it is not too large or it will irritate the healthy skin around the wart.
OR
b) Using 25%-40% salacylic acid paste, scoop a tiny amount on a small spatula, and place it in the hole of the felt.

7. Pack the hole with a tiny wisp of cotton wool and cover it with a bandage or tape.

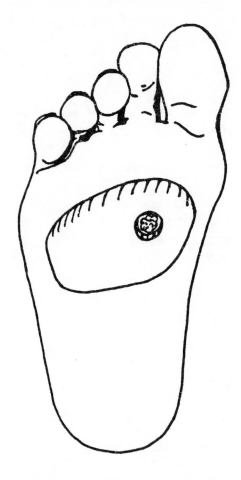

Figure 18: A Cushioned Pad with a Hole around the Plantar Wart

8. Do not wear this pad longer than 12 hours on the first day. After 12 hours or less, remove the pad to check if there is any redness or tenderness. If there is some irritation, wear the pad for a shorter period of time or discontinue the treatment.

9. If everything is fine, continue with the treatment wearing the pad for progressively longer durations, up to five days at a time.

The plaster covering the wart should be changed daily, and if the pad gets wet, then it should also be replaced.

The salicylic acid will destroy the wart slowly, causing the wart tissue to soften and crumble. Each time before replacing the pad, wash your feet in warm water for 10 minutes, and then rub away the soft crumbling skin using a chiropody sponge or a pumice stone. Remember, when you use the chiropody sponge or pumice stone they become contaminated and should not be used for anything else.

Success can be achieved anytime between 4 and 10 weeks of diligent treatment.

The longer the wart has been on your foot, the more stubborn it will be and the longer it will take to be eliminated.

Another foot specialist wrote of a treatment used by one of his patients. The patient rubbed cod liver oil on the wart 4-5 times a day, and eventually it disappeared. It may have worked because of the high vitamin A content in cod liver oil, but I don't know for sure. None of my patients has ever tried this, so I haven't had any first hand experience of its effectiveness, but if you have tried everything else, I guess it's worth a shot.

CLARENCE CRACHETT

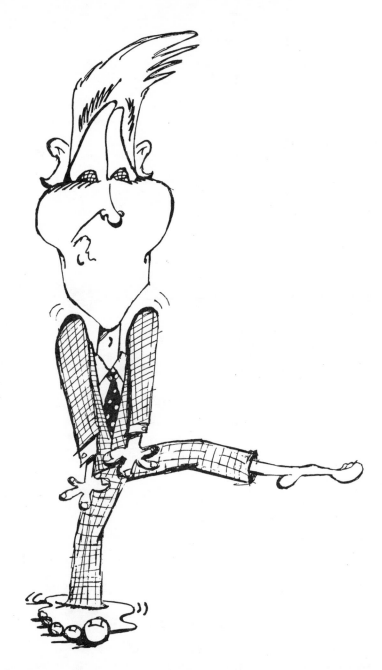

...What looked like well formed arches while he was seated, dropped flat as a pancake when he was bearing his weight

CHAPTER VII

FALLEN ARCHES AND FOOT PAIN

or

How to defeat your "Arch Enemies"

You would think by now I wouldn't be surprised to have a Bunyan or Cratchett referred to my office, but this was different. Clarence Cratchett, Wilemena's younger brother, was not sent to me by one of his relatives, but by his orthopedic surgeon. He went to the orthopedic doctor for pain in his lower back and a very tender spot on his heel. The doctor analyzed the problem and referred him to me.

Clarence Cratchett was a really nice guy with two seemingly unrelated problems that required one solution. The doctor sent over his X-rays which showed nothing unusual in his back, but he did have a nasty spur on his right heel. (See fig. 19)

I examined Clarence's feet while he was sitting on my chair, and outwardly, he had better feet than anyone else I had seen in his family. I gently probed with my fingers at his right heel and found a spot that nearly made Clarence jump right out of the chair.

"That's a heel spur for sure," I thought to myself.

Next, Clarence stood up, and what looked like well formed arches while he was seated, dropped flat as a pancake when he was bearing his weight.

"You've got very weak arches Clarence," I remarked, "and that is causing your heel spur as well as your back pain."

Then I conducted the following test to show him what I had meant. You can do the same thing at home.

1. Remove your shoes and socks and stand with your feet shoulder width apart.

2. Raise the heel of your foot, with the ball of the foot remaining on the ground. Repeat the above procedure with the other foot.

3. If you have a well formed arch while the heel is in the air but it disappears when the heel is on the ground, then you have weak arches.

(Flat feet are something altogether different. If there is no arch while the heel is in the air and no arch while the heel is on the ground, then you have flat feet. This is a problem which should be examined by a foot specialist or orthopedic doctor.)

The solution to Clarence's back problem and heel spur was foot orthotics. These are custom made foot supports that lift the arches, straighten the lower limb and re-balance the muscles in one's back. Although this cured Clarence Cratchett's problem, it's a subject that needs to be discussed in greater detail.

Fallen or weak arches can affect anyone, especially those whose occupations make it necessary to stand most of the day such as waiters, postmen, dentists, factory workers etc. Weak arches cause the entire foot to roll inwards and the heels to angle outward. The bones of the legs rotate with the knees turning in and the hips turning out, causing an imbalance of the muscles of the back.

Common symptoms caused by fallen arches are tired aching feet, legs and back; corns and calluses; ankle swelling; hot burning feet; bunions; bursitis; heel spurs; and poor blood circulation. Your shoes tend to wear out quickly and over a period of time, the pressure on the foot joints can cause osteo-arthritis.

HOME TREATMENT FOR FALLEN ARCHES

or

Forward "M-arch"

1. <u>Simple foot exercises</u> can help strengthen the foot muscles. (see chapter IX).

2. <u>Foot baths</u>: Either contrast foot baths (see page 30) or vibrating heat foot baths (pamper yourself) with a sprinkling of Epsom salts do wonders towards relieving foot aches and stimulating blood circulation.

3. <u>Foot massages</u>: Have your spouse or friend administer a foot massage using a hand held massager or just their fingers. It can be a wonderfully relaxing, soothing, even sensual experience. I used to give my girlfriend foot massages all the time. She is now my wife, so that is what foot massages did for me ... and her.

4. <u>Cushioned insoles</u>: Cushioned insoles placed in your shoes won't help correct fallen arches, but it will help reduce some of the shock and pressure your feet absorb with every step.

5. <u>Custom-made foot supports</u>: You cannot make these yourself at home, but it is the best cure for fallen arches. More information on foot supports is available in chapter X. Briefly, an orthotic will rebalance the foot providing a longer lasting corrective treatment. A well made orthotic will eliminate the problems caused by fallen arches, and the relief you will feel can be overwhelming.

MORE ON HEEL SPURS

"...Which Are Not Just Spur Of The Moment Problems"

A heel spur, which is seen in figure 19, and which showed up on Clarence Cratchett's X-ray, is a growth of calcium around the ligament and muscles of the foot where they attach to the heel bone. It is mainly caused by foot strain. The strain is usually present over a long period of time due to foot problems caused by sports, arthritis, fatigue, poor circulation, foot deformities, excess weight or fallen arches. These problems can cause the arch to elongate which also stretches the ligament attached to the heel. This then creates a small space between the attachment location and the heel bone. The space is filled with calcium, and when you put weight on it, it feels like your stepping on a nail. The area around the spur becomes inflamed, tender and painful. At first it is sore in just one spot, but if it is left unattended, the pain will spread until the entire heel is affected. To avoid this heel pain, your normal walking pattern is altered which can lead to other foot and back problems.

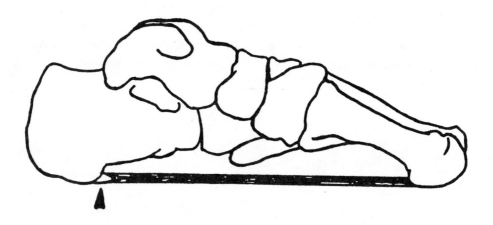

Figure 19: Stretched Plantar Ligaments or Fascia Causing Heel Spur

TREATMENT FOR HEEL SPURS

1. Rest the area and elevate the foot.

2. Apply heat to the sore area. This will stimulate blood circulation and help decrease inflammation.

3. Place a cushioned heel pad in your shoe to reduce the pressure while walking. Instructions for this pad are found on page 97.

If steps 1-3 don't help, then continue to step 4.

4. Ask your family doctor about ultra-sound therapy. Ultra-sound therapy is excellent for the reduction of inflammation. If your doctor does not have an ultra-sound unit, he/she will be able to refer you to a physio therapy clinic that does.

If steps 1-4 haven't helped, and the heel spur has been troubling you for a long time, ask your doctor about a cortisone injection. This treatment will give you temporary instant relief, but let me warn you, it is a very uncomfortable needle.

5. Remove the underlying foot imbalances to support the stretched ligaments and relieve the strain. Custom-made foot orthotics is the best treatment. (See chapter X.)

PART II

COMMON DISEASES WHICH CAN AFFECT THE FEET

CHAPTER VIII

DIABETES

Diabetes is a complicated disease and the causes should be discussed with your own physician. What is important is that you do your bit to keep your blood sugar levels under control by following your doctor's instructions and sticking to your diet.

Why is there so much emphasis put on Foot Care if you are a diabetic? Good question, I'm glad I asked!

Diabetes predominantly affects the small blood vessels in your kidneys, eyes, and feet. When diabetes appears in the body, it can cause many different problems.

1. VASCULAR DISEASE

a) Diabetes disrupts circulation, slowing down the body's natural healing processes. This is the reason it takes a long time for minor cuts to heal. If the minor problem isn't taken care of quickly, it can lead to much bigger problems.

b) The skin becomes thin and shiny, making it more susceptible to abrasions and infections.

c) The skin coloring of the feet and toes change from pink to a bluish purple.

d) The toenails get thick.

2. IMPAIRED PERIPHERAL NERVE FUNCTION

a) The sense of touch or feeling in the legs and feet decreases. This can cause new pressure points on the feet leading to calluses and ulceration.

b) Tingling or pain in the feet and legs are common. Also the skin on the feet and legs gets very dry, and a hot burning sensation may develop.

c) It may become hard to differentiate between hot and cold temperatures.

d) Finally, all sensation in the feet may be lost, including pain. This may sound good, but pain is an important warning sign that something is wrong.

The following was an extreme case, but it shows how quickly a problem can occur in a diabetic foot, and why it is important to examine your feet carefully every day.

I had a patient who spent the day at an amusement park with her grandchildren. She walked around for several hours with a small pebble in her shoe. That night, the first sign she had that something was wrong, occured as she removed her hosiery. Her sock was filled with pus and blood. That little pebble, in a matter of hours, caused a huge ulcer in the bottom of her foot. I'd like to tell you that I performed a miracle and cured her. Unfortunately, there wasn't enough blood circulation to promote healing in her foot, and in order to save her life, the foot had to be amputated.

Knowing what to watch out for, and what to do, will help you give your feet the special care they deserve.

DIABETIC FOOT CARE

1. Wash your feet daily in soapy lukewarm water. Remember to check the temperature with a thermometer, or your wrist or elbow to make sure the water is not too hot!

2. Dry your feet gently with a soft towel using a patting action rather than rubbing. Don't forget to dry underneath and between the toes.

3. After bathing, for dry skin apply lanolin or moisturizing cream. For moist skin, apply rubbing alcohol or dust lightly with talcum powder.

4. Carefully check between the toes, around the nails and on the top and bottom of the feet for cuts, cracks, swelling, bruises, blisters or redness. Use a mirror on the floor to help you or if your eyesight is poor, have someone else check for you.

5. If you locate a problem, bring it to the attention of your doctor or foot specialist.

6. Always cut your nails straight across.

7. Wear only wool or cotton socks.

8. Wear proper fitting shoes, preferably made of leather with a soft insole.

9. Wear soft seamless slippers around the house.

10. Exercise your feet (see Chapter IX).

11. See your doctor regularly.

What you shouldn't do:

1. Do not soak your feet for longer than 10 minutes or your skin will get very dry.

2. Don't walk barefoot.

3. Don't use iodine or a strong antiseptic because they can irritate the skin and the color of iodine may hide any signs of infection (redness) that may occur.

4. Don't cut your own corns or calluses.

5. DON'T EVER USE ANY ACIDS or commercial corn remedies on your feet.

6. Don't wear plastic shoes or sandals.

7. Don't wear nylon hosiery.

8. Don't smoke.

9. Avoid crossing your legs or ankles, (the pressure can reduce circulation).

Things to watch out for:

1. Any color change in your legs or feet.

2. Any injury that doesn't heal or becomes infected.

3. Pain on walking that is relieved by rest.

4. Swelling in the feet or ankles.

5. Unusual coldness, cramping, numbness, tingling or discomfort in your feet.

ARTHRITIS

Arthritis is a disease of the joints and can strike anywhere. No matter where you get it, it is an uncomfortable and painful problem, but when it affects the joints of the feet it can be especially debilitating.

There are two kinds of arthritis, rheumatoid and osteo. Rheumatoid arthritis is a systemic disease that occurs most frequently in young and middle aged people. Osteo arthritis is a degenerative disease that affects many people as they get older. It is this type with which I am most concerned. The symptoms are pain, stiffness and swelling in the joints. It can be caused by many things from a nervous disorder to simple stress. There is no cure at this time, although sometimes it will disappear on its own.

When osteo arthritis affects the feet it can cause fallen arches, bunions, hammer toes, bursitis, heel spurs, corns and calluses.

Treatment consists mainly of relieving the existing symptoms. Your family doctor can prescribe pills to help reduce the pain and inflammation and suggest a nutritional, well balanced diet.

Some additional foot treatments include:

1. Heating lotions containing menthol or camphor, to help relieve the swollen joints.

2. Contrast foot baths (see page 30) or massage foot baths, to stimulate circulation and reduce the aching.

3. Insoles, to cushion your feet as you walk. Sneakers with built-in soft insoles are the best shoes.

4. Foot orthotics to realign the foot, redistribute irregular pressure and cushion the shock on the hip, knees and feet while walking.

5. Cushioned and felt padding to relieve sore painful areas. (See chapter XI.)

GOUT

Ladies you can relax, this is one of those problems that's almost exclusive to men. It was once thought that gout was the disease of kings brought on by an over-indulgence or rich foods, meat and drink. It's not. Good thing it isn't, just think how many people you know would have gout if it were caused by rich foods and drink.

It is a disorder in the body metabolism. The only reason I mention it is because it often appears in the joint of the big toe. Gout can often be confused with other foot problems, but your family doctor can usually diagnose it without any problem. The disorder is relieved by controlling the uric acid level in the body and your doctor can prescribe a drug called "colchicine" to control it.

Foot care simply consists of resting the area to relieve all the pressure.

PART III

CHAPTER IX

FOOT EXERCISES

or

"Have a foot fit for fit feet"

Think. Think hard. Which part of your body is the most cramped and hampered throughout your day? Which part of your body takes the most pressure and abuse? If you guessed "the foot" and by this stage in the book, you had better know the answer, you were right.

Although walking is very good exercise, your shoes will prevent the full range of motions of which your foot muscles are capable. If your feet are to be well toned, foot exercises should be a necessary part of your daily routine. This will help keep your feet strong, and well balanced, with healthy blood circulation. The entire foot exercise routine will take 10-15 minutes and can easily be done while just relaxing or watching TV.

For the following exercises REMOVE YOUR SHOES AND SOCKS and sit on a straight back chair.

REPEAT EACH EXERCISE 10 TIMES

1. Place your foot flat on the floor. Lift the toes and spread them apart. Count to 5 and relax. (You can use your toes to help you count.)

2. a) Place your feet approximately 8 inches apart. Keep your heels on the ground and turn your feet inward so that both big toes try to touch each other.

b) Now turn your feet outward so that the big toes are pulling away from each other.

3. Place a small towel or dishcloth on the floor. Using your toes for gripping, bunch the towel towards you. Feel the pull through each arch.

4. With the legs extended straight out rotate the ankles in large circles, first in one direction, then the other.

5. Stand up. Rise up on your toes and slowly lower your heels.

6. Walk across the room rising high on your toes each time you push off. The more exaggerated the motion, the better the exercise.

7. Walk across the room on your heels, not letting your toes touch the ground.

Enjoy the exercises. They are not very strenuous but are as beneficial as exercises for any other part of your body. Your feet will thank you and you'll feel great.

CHAPTER X

ORTHOTICS

or

"An Uplifting Experience"

I have mentioned "orthotics" or foot supports repeatedly throughout the book. I will now explain why they are an essential part of home foot care.

The aim of an orthotic is to balance the foot so that body weight is carried more evenly by each segment of the foot. This is achieved by exerting gentle, consistent pressure to bring the foot muscles, bones and ligaments back into proper alignment.

Considering the amount of work your feet do daily, it should not be surprising that problems occur. Some 4,000 to 10,000 times a day, the 52 bones, hundreds of ligaments, tendons and muscles of your feet carry your body weight, absorb shock forces. At the same time, your foot joints shift, rotate and then spring back to their original shape. As you get older, your feet, the FOUNDATION OF THE ENTIRE BODY, begin to lose strength, sag, and in many cases, collapse entirely. As with any foundation, a small imbalance can result in severe problems in the rest of the structure.

The need for orthotic correction of the feet is almost as prevalent as the need for optical correction of the eyes. If you have eyesight problems, the need for glasses is obvious, but if you have foot alignment problems, the need for orthotics is not so obvious.

The first signs are usually foot or leg fatigue, calluses, corns, bunions or heel pain. This should indicate to you that the foot joints are improperly balanced, are under too much strain, and are absorbing too much pressure. If nothing is done then the arches will completely flatten, causing back pain, as well as hip and knee pain. Often arthritis will occur, which is not only painful but often disabling.

Okay, I haven't painted a very pretty picture, but relief is available. When a foot specialist determines you need orthotics, he/she will take an impression of your foot similar to the way a dentist takes an impression of your teeth. This negative impression is poured up in plaster of paris, leaving an exact replica of your foot in its corrected position. Finally a custom made orthotic is built right on your "foot statue". When you place your weight on the orthotic, your foot automatically assumes the correct alignment, forcing leg and back muscles into their properly balanced position. The end result over 80% of the time, is the disappearance of foot, leg or back problems.

That is the good news. The bad news is that a foot doctor charges approximately $300.00 or more for a pair of orthotics.

So here we are, I've told you all these wonderful things about orthotics, but now you're depressed because they are too darn expensive. Well if you are still interested, and you should be, you will be pleased to know that I have made a very special arrangement with a large orthotic laboratory. They have agreed to provide my readers with the same high quality orthotics available from doctors, for less than half the price using a new innovative technique. (Check the coupon at the back of the book).

PART 4

CHAPTER XI

HOW TO CONSTRUCT FOOT PADS

How often have you told yourself, "when your feet hurt you hurt all over" !

For someone with foot pain there is no truer statement in the whole world. But now you have a choice. No longer will you have to put up with that painful corn, callus, heel spur or pressure spot. It is within your power to make yourself a simple pad to relieve the pain - immediately!

Foot pads can be made from different materials. The best pad for redistributing pressure is 1/4" felt, with an adhesive backing. For cushioning sore spots, foam with an adhesive backing is best. These are the two materials discussed in the instructions for making your own foot pads. Some drugstores carry these materials in their footcare sections.

You will learn how to make pads that can stick on your feet, or can be removed from and replaced on your feet repeatedly.

Stick-on pads are best if your foot is very sore. This kind of pad will not move around once it is placed on the foot, and will accurately cushion or deflect pressure away from the sore area. Generally a stick-on pad will last three to five days before a new one must be applied. It tends to lose its effectiveness more quickly if the pad gets wet.

Replaceable pads, like the name suggests, can be reused many times. When you bathe or go to bed the pad is removed, and reapplied when you begin weightbearing. A replaceable pad can last up to several weeks before a new one is needed.

Replaceable pads may move around on your foot, depending on how well the straps are made. Sometimes it may not be as accurate as a stick-on pad. A replaceable pad just requires a little more skill to construct, but with a little practice can be mastered easily.

A FEW HINTS TO REMEMBER
WHILE CUTTING PADS

1. When you attempt to construct a pad for the first time, it is best to use a piece of cardboard as a model, instead of felt. This way, if you do make an error, no felt or cushioned padding will be wasted.

2. After you've completed a replaceable pad or applied a stick-on pad, sprinkle a little talcum powder over the pad. This will reduce friction and help the pad last longer.

3. Try to keep your pads dry. Getting them wet may reduce the effectiveness of the pad. Some of my patients have washed their replaceable pads by hand, and they were still useful. So, if you wish, try it once. If you ruin the pad don't do it again, if not, well . . . go for it.

4. Don't hurry. Making a pad is similiar to cutting out paper dolls, so relax and have fun. You are being creative, and have nothing to lose but your foot pain!

For those of you who have difficulty finding the felt or cushioned padding, or any of the materials necessary to cut your own foot pads, send the coupon at Ithe back of "SECRETS TO HOME FOOT CARE", requesting information on the "complete kit for cutting foot pads at home".

SOLE METATARSAL PADS

A. DEFLECTIVE METATARSAL PAD

This pad is the most common pad constructed by a foot specialist.It can be useful for relieving pressure from calluses across the ball of the foot. It also can help reduce pain across the top of your foot.

1. Feel the bottom of your foot and find the heads of your metatarsal bones. Your metatarsals are the long bones in the foot which attach to your toes. Do this by flexing your toes up and down and feel the bone jut out. If it will help mark the heads of the bones with lipstick or a pen. (See fig.20)

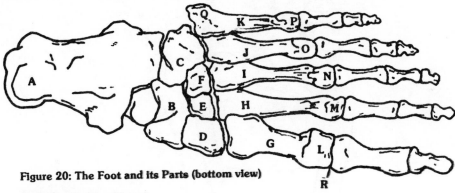

Figure 20: The Foot and its Parts (bottom view)

A: Calcaneus (heel bone)
B: Navicular
C: Cuboid
D: Medial (inner) Cuniform
E: Middle Cuniform
F: Lateral (outer) Cuniform
G: 1st Metatarsal bone
H: 2nd Metatarsal bone
I: 3rd Metatarsal bone
J: 4th Metatarsal bone
K: 5th Metatarsal bone
L: Head of the 1st Metatarsal bone
M: Head of the 2nd Metatarsal bone
N: Head of the 3rd Metatarsal bone
O: Head of the 4th Metatarsal bone
P: Head of the 5th Metatarsal bone
Q: Base of the 5th Metatarsal bone
R: 1st Metatarso-phalangeal Joint (where bunions occur)

2. Using 1/4" felt padding, cut the pad so that the front of the pad follows the heads of your metatarsals. The length of the pad extends to the base of your fifth metatarsal bone. Feel the side of your foot and you will easily find the spot. The width of the pad should extend from the head of your first metatarsal to the head of your 5th metatarsal.

3. Once you've got the correct shape, with a sharp pair of scissors, angle or level the edges of the pad so there is a gradual declining from the pad to the skin.

At the front of the pad, angle the edge so that the thickest part of the pad is directly behind the heads of the metatarsals.
At the back of the pad, angle back 1/4 to 1/3 the length of the pad.

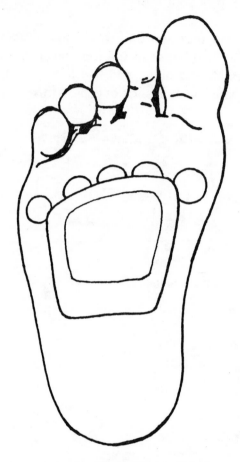

Figure 21: A Sole Metatarsal Pad

At both sides cut the corners of the pad.

4. Pull off the backing of the pad and place on the foot.

5. Cover the pad with zinc oxide 2" wide tape or other kinds of foot care tapes and sprinkle with a light coating of talcum powder.

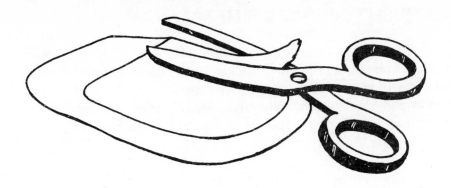

Figure 22: A Sole Metatarsal Pad with Correctly Angled Edges

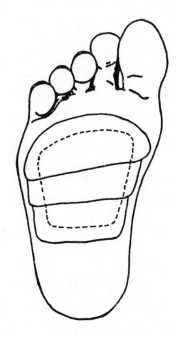

Figure 23: A Sole Metatarsal Pad Adhered to the Foot with the First Strap of 2" Tape

6. When you step down on the pad you will notice the heads of your metatarsal bones will rise upwards and your toes will move downwards. Now you have transferred pressure from the heads of the metatarsal bones onto the toes where some of the weight belongs.

B. CUSHIONING SOLE METATARSAL PAD

For those who have very little fat on the bottom of your foot, and it feels as if you are walking on bones all the time, you just need cushioning over the heads of your metatarsals. Using cushioned padding instead of felt, follow the same instructions as in pad 'A'. The only difference is that you must extend the front portion of the pad so that the thickness of the cushion is directly over your metatarsal heads instead of behind them. .

C. SOLE METATARSAL PAD WITH A "U"

This is used for a severe corn or callus directly over the head of the 2nd, 3rd or 4th metatarsal head. This kind of a problem is usually a sign of a dropped metatarsal bone which is absorbing too much pressure. (See fig. 10)

1. Using 1/4" felt padding, cut the pad exactly the same as in pad 'A', with the following two changes:

a) Cut the pad slightly wider so that the width goes to the outside of the 1st and 5th metatarsal heads.

b. Cut a small "U" around the painful metatarsal head as in fig 24.

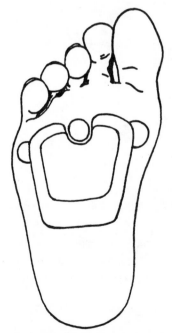

Figure 24: A Sole Metatarsal Pad with a Center Cutout

D. SOLE METATARSAL PAD WITH A SINGLE CORNER CUTOUT

This is used for a corn, callus or painful 1st or 5th metatarsal head. This kind of problem is usually a sign of an imbalanced foot with the front of the foot tilting toward the inside or outside of the foot.

1. Using 1/4" felt padding cut the pad the same as pad 'A' with the following changes:

a) Cut the pad wider so that the edge of the pad on the side of the sore metatarsal extends to the edge of the foot.

b) Cut off the corner of the pad around the metatarsal head as in fig. 25.

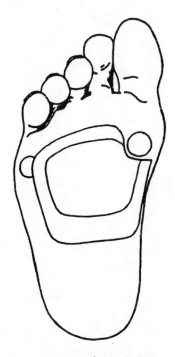

Figure 25: A Sole Metatarsal Pad with a Single Corner Cutout

E. SOLE METATARSAL PAD WITH DOUBLE CORNER CUTOUTS

This is used for a corn or callus on both the 1st and 5th metatarsal heads. It is usually a sign of a hypermobile foot with the 2nd, 3rd and 4th metatarsals absorbing little or no body weight at all.

1. Using 1/4" felt padding cut the pad the same as pad 'D', with the following addition:

a) Extend both edges of the pad to the sides of the foot and then cut both corners of the pad as seen in fig. 26

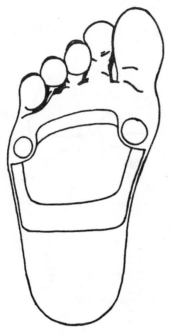

Figure 26: A Sole Metatarsal Pad with a Double Corner Cutout

REPLACEABLE SOLE METATARSAL PADS - ALL KINDS

1. Cut the pad the same as a stick-on pad, except the felt or cushion padding should be touching the skin and the sticky peel-back paper facing out.

2. Measure a piece of elastic strapping around your foot. Peel the paper off the back of the pad and place the strapping approximately three quarters of the way to the end of the pad. (See fig. 27). The strap should not be too loose or the pad

will slip, or too tight which could cut off blood circulation. It should be comfortably snug.

3. Cut a strip of 1" zinc oxide tape and fold it in half so it will stick to itself. Use this as your toe loop. Loop the tape over the three middle toes and extend it to the sticky side of the pad.

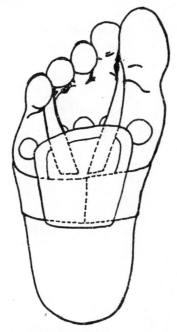

Figure 27: A Replaceable Sole Metatarsal Pad with an elastic strap around the foot and a tape

4. Remove the pad from your foot and cover the back of it with moleskin or strips of 2" zinc oxide tape. Apply a light sprinkling of talc powder on both sides of the pad.

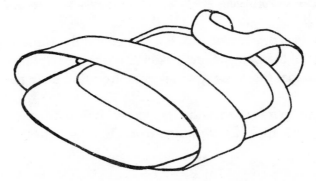

Figure 28: A Top View of a Completed Replaceable Sole Metatarsal Pad

SOLE SHAFT PAD

A shaft pad is an easier pad to construct than a Sole Metatarsal Pad and is used when you have a callus or corn over one sore metatarsal head. It will lift the single metatarsal relieving the pressure. This pad cannot be made as a replaceable pad and is an alternative to the Sole Metatarsal Pad with a 'U' or 'Corner Cutout'.

1. Using 1/4" felt padding, cut a rectangle with the width slightly wider than the metatarsal and the length extending from the head of the metatarsal to the base of the 5th metatarsal as seen in fig. 29.

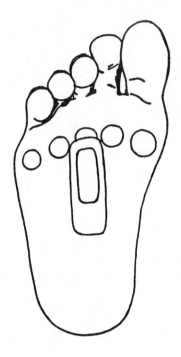

Figure 29: Correct Positioning of a Sole Shaft Pad for the Third Metatarsal Head

2. To angle the edges of the pad, trim the corners off the sides, trim the front so that the thickness of the pad is directly behind the metatarsal head, and trim the end of the pad so that there is a gradual slope from the thick pad to your foot.

3. Stick the pad on your foot ensuring the thickest part is directly behind the sore metatarsal head, and apply 2" wide zinc oxide to tape adhere the pad to your foot.

4. Apply a light sprinkling of talcum powder over the pad.

PADS FOR PAINFUL HEELS

As the name suggests the following are pads for those with sore or tender heels.

A. HEEL PAD

1. Using 1/4" cushion padding this pad can be adhered to the foot but it is esier to stick it right in the shoes.

2. Cut out a piece of cardboard that fits exactly around the heel of the shoe extending to where the arch meets the heel bone.

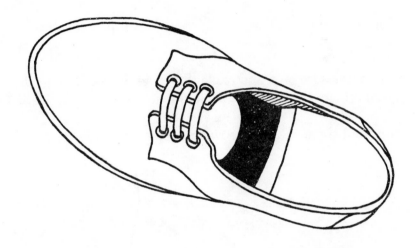

Figure 30: A Heel Cushion Pad inside the Shoe

Using the cardboard as your guide, cut a cushioned pad to fit in the heel angling the area closest to the arch.

B. HEEL SPUR PAD

Cut the same as a heel pad with the following change:

Find the exact sore spot on your heel and color it with lipstick. (If you don't want lipstick on your heel cover it with a piece of tape then dab the lipstick on the tape.)

Place the cardboard in your shoe and walk around the room.

The lipstick will leave its mark on the cardboard and that is the exact area you cut out to relieve the pressure on the heel.

Note: When cutting heel pads always make them for both feet so that one leg isn't raised higher than the other.

BUNION PADS

A bunion pad is used to deflect pressure away from a sore on the 1st or 5th toe joint at the side of your foot.

This problem is usually caused from shoe pressure, so if you can, wear wider shoes.

1. Using 1/4" felt or cushion padding cut an oval shaped pad which will cover the joint entirely

2. a) Cut a hole over the sore area and angle the edges as seen in fig. 31.
   b) Cut a crescent around the area and angle the edges as seen in fig. 32.

3. Cover with tape and sprinkle talcum powder over the pad.

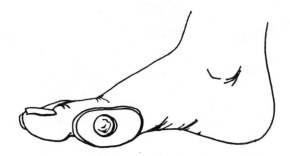

Figure **31: An Oval Bunion Pad**

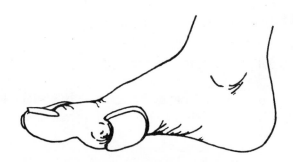

Figure **32: A Crescent Bunion Pad**

SECRETS TO HOME FOOT CARE

CORN PADS

PADS FOR CORNS ON THE TOPS OF TOES

A. HORSESHOE CRESCENT PAD

A horseshoe crescent pad is used to protect against corns on the tops of the toes.

1. Using 1/4" felt padding, cut the pad so that it fits directly behind the sore area with a small hole around the corn.

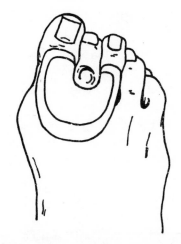

**Figure 33: A Horseshoe Crescent Pad
Around a Corn on the Top of the 2nd Toe**

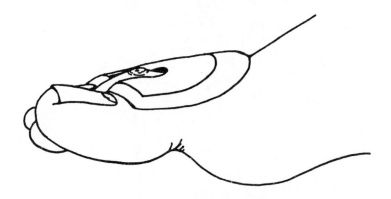

**Figure 34: A Side View of a Horseshoe Crescent Pad
around the Corn at the Top of the 2nd Toe**

2. Angle the sides of the pad.

3. Cover with the pad with tape so it will not move.

REPLACEABLE PADS FOR THE TOPS OF THE TOES

This pad is useful for corns on the tops of your toes as well as toes that flex upwards and rub against your shoes.

1. Using felt or cushioned padding, cut the same as the above pad with the sticky side facing out.

2. Cut a small piece of elastic strapping to fit around the toe.

3. Cover the pad with moleskin or tape.

4. Apply a light sprinkling of talcum powder.

This pad can be cut larger to protect 2 or 3 toes.

B. OVAL PAD WITH A HOLE

This pad is a variation of the previous pad.

1. Using 1/4" felt padding, cut an oval with a hole over sore area.

2. Angle the edges.

3. Cover with tape and add a light sprinkling of talcum powder.

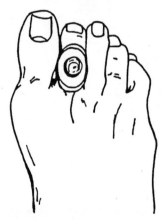

Figure 35: An Oval Pad with a Hole for a Corn on the Top of the 2nd Toe

SECRETS TO HOME FOOT CARE

TOE PROPS

This pad is useful for raising the toes so that the corns at the tips of the toes will disappear, or to help straighten out curved toes.

1. Cut two pieces of felt the width of the toes which are to be raised off the ground.

2. Stick the two pads together and angle them so that the felt will fit under the toes and raise them up as in fig. 36.

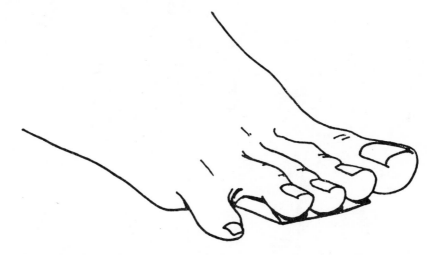

Figure 36: A Side View of a Toe Prop under the 2nd, 3rd, and 4th Toes

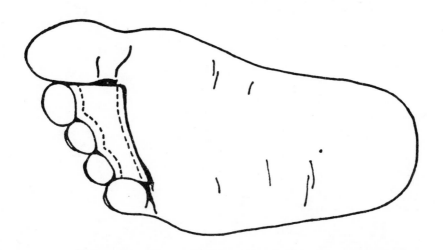

Figure 37: Bottom View of a Toe Prop under the 2nd, 3rd and 4th Toes

REPLACEABLE TOE PROP

1. Everything is the exact same as above except cut a piece of elastic strapping which fits around the toes BEFORE sticking the two pieces of felt together.

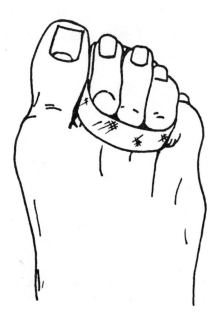

Figure 38: Top View of a Replaceable Toe Prop with an Elastic Strap

TOE WEDGE PAD FOR CORNS BETWEEN THE TOES

When a corn appears between the toes it can be sooo painful, but it is sooo easy to fix. By keeping the area between the toes dry, and separating the toes, the 'rubbing pressure' that caused the corn will stop, and the corn will quickly disappear.

1. Using cushion or felt padding, cut a wedge at the toe webbing and round the pad at the front. Place the pad between the sore toes as in fig. 39.

2. Adding a hole where the corn is situated will help relieve even more of the painful pressure.

3. Apply a light sprinkling of talcum powder.

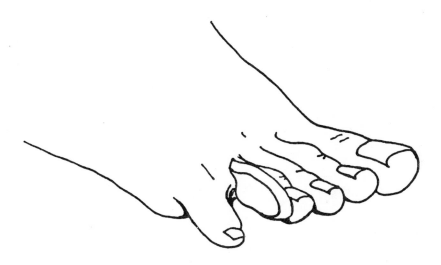

Figure 39: A Toe Wedge Pad for a Corn between the 4th and 5th Toes

REPLACEABLE TOE WEDGE

1. Cut the pad the same as above.

2. Add an elastic strap that sticks to the adhesive side of the padding, and fits snugly around the toe. (Always fit the strap around the 2nd, 3rd or 4th toes, because it will sit better in your shoes.)

3. Cover the sticky side of the padding with tape or moleskin, or another piece of padding.

4. Apply a light sprinkling of talcum powder.

AFTERWORD

I hope you have enjoyed "SECRETS TO HOME FOOT CARE", (except that now they are no longer secrets), and that this book has helped you defeat da problems of de feet!

As mentioned earlier, I will be glad to answer any personal questions - as long as they're about your feet.

In the meantime, kick off your shoes and pamper your feet.

HOW TO PAMPER YOUR FEET
AT THE END OF A LONG HARD DAY

1. Remove your shoes and socks.

2. Take a few deep breaths and let the air out slowly.

3. Soak your feet in warm sudsy water for about 10 minutes. If you have a foot-bath/vibrator, use it.

4. Dry your feet thoroughly with a towel.

5. Stand on your towel and gather it up using your toes.

6. Next, alternate standing on your heels then on your toes. Do this 10-20 times.

7. Massage your feet:
a) First rub a stimulating or moisturizing cream on your feet.
b) Grab your toes and rotate them inward and outward five times.
c) Using the flat of your hand, your fist or your thumb, massage each sole from your heel to the toes and back again. Do this for as long as you wish. It's even better if someone else does it for you.

Experiment with your feet. Pull gently on each toe, rub the top of your foot - whatever feels good!

Now that you, your feet and your whole body feel better, -- get out of neutral and get on with your activities.

And remember...

Your feet need to give you a lifetime of support.
Treat them right and you'll always be an upstanding citizen - or a least a citizen who stands up!!

Well folks, here it is. Throughout the book I have encouraged you to remember your questions until you reached the end.

This is it! Your chance to receive additional information or a confidential answer to your specific problem.

Complete the following coupon, enclose a self-addressed stamped envelope, and send it to the following address:

in the U.S.A.
Footsaver Publishing
908 Niagara Falls Blvd.
N. Tonawanda, NY 14120-2060

in Canada
Footsaver Publishing
5334 Yonge St., Suite 1403
Toronto, Ont., M2N 6M2

please print

- -

[   ]   YES!   I Have a question I want J. Schneider to answer for me.

[   ]   YES!   I have included a self addressed stamped envelope.

MY QUESTION IS:

_____

_____

_____

_____

_____

(use an additional page if necessary)

Even if you do not have a question, you may receive more FREE information on any of the following.

[   ]   YES!   Please send me information on:

[   ]   *The Home Footcare Kit:* This includes felt padding, cushion padding, elastic strapping, tape, and tubefoam.

[   ]   *Customized Orthotics:* Foot supports which will rebalance your feet, and realign the muscles in your legs and back.

[   ]   *Perspiring Feet & Foot Odor:* Preparations and treatments for problem sweaty and smelly feet.

[   ]   *Foot Creams:* Creams for removing callus, moisturizing dry feet, and cooling hot burning feet.

[   ]   *Foot Care Instruments:* Including nail clippers, files, pumice stones, and more.

[   ]   *Assorted General Footcare Products:* A full line of products to soothe and pamper your feet.

NAME: _____

ADDRESS: _____

CITY: _____

STATE/PROV.: _____ POSTAL CODE: _____